Ultrasound-Guided Regional Anesthesia

A Practical Approach to Peripheral Nerve Blocks and Perineural Catheters

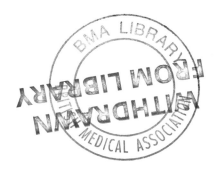

Ultrasound-Guided Regional Anesthesia

A Practical Approach to Peripheral Nerve Blocks and Perineural Catheters

Fernando L. Arbona

Babak Khabiri

John A. Norton

Illustrated by Charles Hamilton and Kelly Warniment

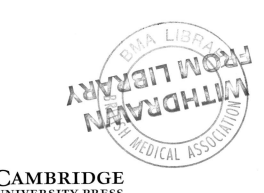
CAMBRIDGE
UNIVERSITY PRESS

CAMBRIDGE UNIVERSITY PRESS
Cambridge, New York, Melbourne, Madrid, Cape Town, Singapore,
São Paulo, Delhi, Dubai, Tokyo, Mexico City

Cambridge University Press
The Edinburgh Building, Cambridge CB2 8RU, UK

Published in the United States of America by
Cambridge University Press, New York

www.cambridge.org
Information on this title: www.cambridge.org/9780521515788

© Cambridge University Press 2011

First published 2011

Printed in the United Kingdom at the University Press, Cambridge

A catalog record for this publication is available from the British Library

Library of Congress Cataloging-in-Publication Data

Arbona, Fernando L.
    Ultrasound-guided regional anesthesia : a practical approach to
peripheral nerve blocks and perineural catheters / Fernando L. Arbona,
Babak Khabiri, John A. Norton.
        p. ; cm.
    Includes bibliographical references and index.
    ISBN 978-0-521-51578-8 (Hardback)
1. Conduction anesthesia.   2. Operative ultrasonography.
3. Ultrasonic imaging.   I. Khabiri, Babak.   II. Norton, John A.,
1971–   III. Title.
    [DNLM: 1. Nerve Block–methods.   2. Anesthesia, Local–methods.
3. Anesthetics, Local.   4. Catheterization, Peripheral–methods.
5. Peripheral Nerves–ultrasonography.   6. Ultrasonography,
Interventional–methods.   WO 300 A666u 2010]
    RD84.A73 2010
    617.9′64–dc22
                                                        2010008737

ISBN 978-0-521-51578-8 Hardback

Additional resources for this publication at
www.cambridge.org/arbona

Fernando L. Arbona
This book is dedicated to my wife, Melissa, and my three beautiful daughters, Olivia, Sophia, and Mia, who provide me with the love, support, and inspiration that help me in all of life's endeavors.

Babak Khabiri
For my parents Badi Khabiri and Mahin Raz Khabiri who instilled in us a love for learning and helping others; and my three older brothers Ramin, Shahriar, and Hooman who showed me the way.

John A. Norton
I would like to thank my wife Kavitha for always providing a foundation of loving support in my professional endeavors, and our beautiful children, J. P., Meera, and Joshua for their daily inspiration.

Contents

Free access website at **www.cambridge.org/arbona** containing numerous ultrasound loops and video clips showing nerve block and perineural catheter techniques being performed.

Preface

Ultrasound guidance in regional anesthesia provides real-time imaging during the placement of nerve blocks and perineural catheters, improving patient comfort, decreasing many procedure times, and revealing valuable anatomic information, which may enhance patient safety. It therefore comes as no surprise that the use of ultrasound in regional anesthesia continues to grow in popularity, opening new doors to physicians in their practice where barriers may have once existed. As regional anesthesiologists, we have written this text for residents, fellows, and staff physicians desiring to learn and begin incorporating the use of ultrasound into the scope of their busy practices.

This book introduces the use of ultrasound technology for the placement of peripheral nerve blocks and perineural catheters. Our goal in writing this text was to provide an easy-to-read source of information with particular attention to the steps and detail involved with ultrasound imaging, as well as block and catheter placement.

We have organized the text into four major sections, beginning with chapters to introduce basic concepts in regional anesthesia including local anesthetics, ultrasound physics and imaging, as well as anatomy. The chapter on local anesthetics is written to convey basic pharmacologic concepts about the medications commonly used in peripheral nerve blocks. Multiple, more in-depth sources other than this text are available for review. Our intention here is to introduce agents common to the practice of regional anesthesia with concise, retainable information for anesthesia providers.

The introduction to ultrasound is divided into two separate chapters (Chapters 2 and 3). The first of these chapters discusses basic principles of ultrasound physics and imaging, while the second covers the current utilization of this technology in a regional anesthesia setting. An in-depth discussion of probe manipulation, image optimization, and troubleshooting techniques is provided. For the beginner, these chapters are important, and they are written to be easy to follow with information and nomenclature that will become commonplace as you implement ultrasound into your practice.

The middle sections of the text (Sections 2 and 3) discuss the placement of ultrasound-guided single-shot regional blocks that can be routinely used in most busy anesthesia practices. Section 2 focuses on upper extremity peripheral nerve blocks, while Section 3 turns to blocks of the lower extremity. Each chapter is introduced with a discussion of pertinent anatomy in the block region. An understanding of anatomical structures and relationships is key when ultrasound imaging is undertaken during scanning and block placement. All chapters provide specific instruction on block selection and set up, needle positioning, local anesthetic injection, and troubleshooting.

Section 4 includes chapters detailing the practical placement and positioning of continuous perineural catheters under ultrasound guidance. We feel this is a unique feature of this text.

While we do summarize procedures for quick, easy reference, portions of each procedural chapter are written as if the instructor were there performing the block with you. Further, our "Key points" or "Additional considerations" paragraphs outlined within the text of each chapter are there to provide additional hints, reminders, or instructions, which may improve block success or enhance safety in your practice.

Much of the information in these chapters we draw from our own experience as instructors at a major academic medical center and a fast-paced ambulatory setting. The "Authors' clinical practice" sections highlight our own personal practice and opinions regarding topics covered in the preceding chapter. We developed these discussions as a "see how we do it" section for quick, easy reference at the end of each chapter. These are the answers to questions we are often asked when teaching these techniques. Though we do not attest that this is always the preferred or best way to achieve a specific desired result, we have found the points made in these discussions to be most efficacious in our own practice.

For those new to ultrasound in regional anesthesia and a particular block approach, we find the best use of this book is in review of the detail-oriented sections prior to undertaking new techniques. Summary sections within each chapter can then be referred to later for quick and easy review. And just as we teach our residents, we advocate becoming proficient with single-shot peripheral nerve blocks utilizing ultrasound before attempting perineural catheter placement.

This book was written to organize and convey to others the instruction we use and teach in our daily practice. If you are interested in picking up an ultrasound probe to assist with your next peripheral nerve block, this book was written for you.

Acknowledgments

This book would not have been possible without the support of the Ohio State University and the Department of Anesthesiology. We have come to recognize that teaching is a two-way process and the more we teach the more we learn. As such, this book is a product of our daily interactions with residents who over the years challenged us to become better educators and clinicians. We would like to thank the numerous surgeons at the Ohio State University Hospital East who have been so supportive of our regional anesthesia program and our efforts to provide the best and the most advanced care to the patients we encounter.

We would like to thank Dr. Charles Hamilton for his work in providing the anatomical illustrations used in this textbook and to Kelly Warniment for her physics diagrams.

Last, but not least, we have to acknowledge the invaluable help and guidance of Laurah Carlson, "the pain nurse", whose hard work and dedication improves the lives of all those who come under her care.

1

Pharmacology: local anesthetics and additives

Introduction

An understanding of basic local anesthetic pharmacology is essential prior to safe and effective placement of any regional block. Numerous pharmacology texts and literature sources are available describing similarities and differences with regard to onset time, duration, selective motor and/or sensory blockade, tissue penetration, and toxic profile. The goal of this chapter is to provide a brief overview of the more common local anesthetics used in performing peripheral nerve blocks.

To introduce the mechanism of local anesthetic action, the chapter begins with a brief review of nerve electrophysiology. A short discussion on local anesthetic structure is then covered followed by key points regarding pharmacologic properties of individual agents commonly used in peripheral nerve blocks. Local anesthetic toxicity and its management are reviewed, and the chapter concludes with a discussion of local anesthetic additives for peripheral nerve blocks.

Nerve electrophysiology

One of the basic ways peripheral nerve fibers can be grouped is based on the presence or absence of a myelin sheath surrounding the nerve axon (Figure 1.1). Myelin, composed mostly of lipid, provides a layer of insulation around the nerve axon when present. Most nerves within the peripheral nervous system are myelinated (except C-fibers, which are un-myelinated) with variations in size and function. The largest myelinated nerves (A-alpha) are 12 to 20 micrometers thick and are involved with motor and proprioceptive functioning. In comparison, the smallest myelinated (A-delta) and un-myelinated (C-fibers) are around 1 to 2 micrometers or less in diameter and play a role in transmission of pain and temperature sensation.

Impulses travel along the un-myelinated portions of nerves in waves of electrical activity called action potentials. Nerves without myelin propagate action potentials in a continuous wave of electrical activity along the nerve's axon.

Action potentials are spread a bit differently, and faster, in myelinated nerves. Nerves containing myelin have small un-myelinated sections along the nerve's axon called nodes of Ranvier (Figure 1.1). Instead of traveling continuously down the axon, impulses jump from one node of Ranvier to the next, a concept known as saltatory conduction. Saltatory conduction allows action potentials to spread faster in myelinated nerves.

Nerve cells maintain a resting potential gradient with extracellular fluid of approximately $-70\,mV$ to $-90\,mV$. This resting gradient exists as positively charged sodium ions (Na^+) are actively pumped out of the cell in exchange for potassium ions (K^+) across transmembrane proteins via a Na/K ATPase. In addition to the active transfer of Na^+ out, K^+ flows out passively from the cell's inner cytoplasm to the extracellular space. This net flow of positively charged ions out of the cell's interior at rest leads to a consistent negative resting potential gradient across the nerve cell axonal membrane.

Action potentials are formed as a result of positive fluctuations in this resting potential gradient. These fluctuations occur with changes in Na^+ concentration and direction of flow across the nerve cell membrane. Stimulation of the nerve leads to activation of Na^+ channels spanning the nerve cell's membrane, allowing Na^+ to now flow *into* the cell's interior. As Na^+ enters the cell, the negative transmembrane potential difference becomes more positive. At a cellular threshold of approximately $-60\,mV$, additional Na^+ channels are activated, leading to rapid depolarization of the nerve cell followed by action potential formation. The nerve cell membrane depolarizes and

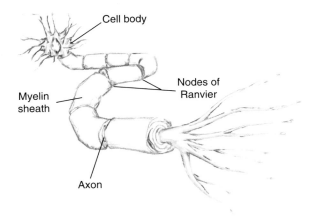

Figure 1.1 Nodes of Ranvier on a myelinated nerve fiber.

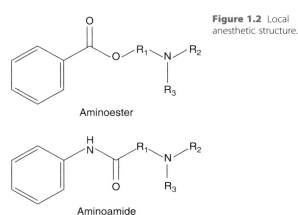

Figure 1.2 Local anesthetic structure.

rises to a potential difference of +20 mV before the transmembrane Na^+ channels become inactivated. The resting membrane potential difference is ultimately restored by the active Na/K ATPase and passive leakage of K^+ back out of the cell.

Additional considerations

Local anesthetics exert their effect at the inner portion of transmembrane Na^+ channel proteins. By reversibly binding these channels, depolarization of the nerve axon is prevented.

Local anesthetic pharmacology

Local anesthetic structure and classification

Local anesthetics are composed of lipophilic and hydrophilic ends connected by an intermediate chain.

The "head" of the molecule is an aromatic ring structure and the most lipophilic portion of the molecule, while the "tail" portion is a tertiary (neutral) or quaternary (charged) amine derivative. The intermediate carbon chain, which forms the body of the molecule, is connected to the amine portion typically by an amide or ester linkage (Figure 1.2). It is this association that is used to classify the commonly used local anesthetic agents as either an ester or an amide.

Local anesthetic pharmacodynamics

Local anesthetic ionization and pKA

Local anesthetics are weak bases and, by definition, poorly soluble and only partially ionized in aqueous solution. For stability, preparations of local anesthetics are stored as hydrochloride salts with an acidic pH ranging from 3 to 6.

It has long been felt an agent's pKa correlates closely to the speed of onset for a particular local anesthetic. There are, however, a number of factors that may be associated with onset time for these agents, especially when used in peripheral nerve blocks. Such factors include lipid solubility of the anesthetic, the type of block and proximity of anesthetic injection to the nerve, the type and size of nerve fibers blocked, and the degree of local anesthetic ionization.

It is the relationship between the agent's pKa and surrounding pH that relates to the degree of ionization for the drug (Table 1.1). The pKa is the pH at which the agent exists as a 50:50 mixture of ionized and free base (non-ionized) molecules. In other words, these agents exist in a continuum of ionized and neutral form in solution with the balance point at the agent's pKa. At physiologic pH, the balance favors the ionized form since those clinically relevant local anesthetics used in peripheral nerve blocks have a pKa in excess of the pH of extracellular fluid. But the lower a drug's pKa in physiologic solution, the more drug is available in the neutral form.

It is the neutral form of the drug that passes into and through the nerve cell membrane. The greater amount of drug in the neutral form available to pass into the nerve cell, one might surmise, the faster the onset. While this theory is commonly accepted, it is not without exception, as is the case with chloroprocaine (pKa 8.7). Among the amide local anesthetics, however, this relationship seems to hold true.

Once inside the nerve cell, it is the ionized form of the local anesthetic that attaches to the

Table 1.1 Pharmacokinetic and pharmacodynamic differences between common ester and amide local anesthetics used in peripheral nerve blocks

Agent	Type	Pot	pKa	%PB	Dur	Met
2-Chloroprocaine (Nesacaine®)	E	Low	8.7	–	S	Pl esterase
Lidocaine (Xylocaine®)	A	Int	7.9	64.3	Int	Hepatic
Mepivacaine (Carbocaine®)	A	Low	7.6	77.5	Int	Hepatic
Bupivacaine (Marcaine®/Sensorcaine®)	A	High	8.1	95.6	L	Hepatic
Levobupivacaine	A	High	8.1	>97	L	Hepatic
Ropivacaine (Naropin®)	A	Int	8.1	94	L	Hepatic

Notes: A = amide type; E = ester type; Pot = potency; %PB = percentage protein binding; Dur = approximate duration in peripheral nerve blockade; S = short; Int = intermediate; L = long; Met = metabolism; Pl esterase = plasma esterase.

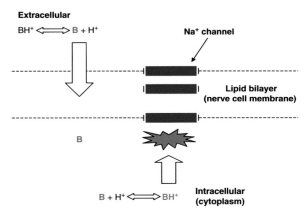

Figure 1.3 Non-ionized local anesthetic crossing the nerve cell membrane to affect intracellular portion of sodium channel as ionized drug.

internal portion of the Na$^+$ channel to exert the drug's effect (Figure 1.3).

Potency/lipophilicity

Lipid solubility of local anesthetic agents is a major determinant of drug potency. Lipid solubility is often quantified by use of a partition coefficient. The partition coefficient for a particular agent is a ratio of the un-ionized concentration of the drug between two solvents: an aqueous (ionized) solvent (e.g., water) and some non-ionized, hydrophobic solvent (e.g., hexane). In general, as the partition coefficient increases, so too does the agent's lipid solubility. Ultimately, the more lipid soluble an agent, the greater it's potency (Table 1.1).

Protein binding

Plasma proteins avidly bind to local anesthetics in circulation, essentially inactivating the drug. It is the free, unbound form of the drug that is active. Serum alpha 1-acid glycoprotein binds local anesthetics with high affinity along with serum albumin. As the drug is absorbed from the site of administration, serum proteins bind to the free drug in circulation until serum protein stores are saturated.

The affinity of local anesthetic agents for protein molecules has been correlated with the duration of anesthetic effect, though a number of other pharmacologic and physiologic factors are ultimately involved (Table 1.1).

Drug effect

Local anesthetics are capable of blocking nerve action potentials by reversibly binding to the intracellular portion of sodium channel proteins within nerve cell membranes.

To exert this effect, the un-ionized, neutral form of the anesthetic crosses into and through the nerve cell membrane (Figure 1.3). Once inside the cell, the anesthetic is ionized and binds to the inner portion of transmembrane sodium channels. By attatching to the sodium channels within the nerve cell membrane, local anesthetics prevent depolarization of the nerve cell, reducing action potential formation.

Local anesthetic metabolism

Amide local anesthetics are predominantly broken down by the liver. The rate of metabolism depends primarily on liver blood flow and the particular agent used, as some variability does exist. In general, lidocaine and mepivacaine tend to be more rapidly metabolized than ropivacaine and bupivacaine.

Ester local anesthetics are rapidly metabolized by plasma pseudo-cholinesterase. As such, their metabolism may be prolonged in patients with severe liver dysfunction, pseudo-cholinesterase deficiency, or atypical pseudo-cholinesterase. While the metabolites of ester local anesthetics are inactive, they can rarely be allergenic as para-aminobenzoic acid (PABA) has been implicated in allergic reactions to ester agents.

Commonly used local anesthetics for peripheral nerve blocks

2-Chloroprocaine

2-Chloroprocaine (Nesacaine®) is an amino-ester local anesthetic that was first marketed in the 1950s. The drug has a rapid onset and short duration when used for peripheral nerve blockade, and is a popular choice for cases of short duration where postoperative analgesia is not a concern. The agent is available in 1%, 2% (preservative-free), and 3% (preservative-free) concentrations. Use of 3% 2-chloroprocaine in volumes of 20 to 30 ml may yield 1.5 to 3 hours of surgical anesthesia with a very low toxicity profile relative to commonly used amide local anesthetics due to its extremely rapid metabolism in the plasma.

Lidocaine

Lidocaine (Xylocaine®) was the first synthetic amino-amide local anesthetic developed (1940s) and remains one of the most popular agents available today. Used in peripheral nerve blocks, the drug's onset, duration, and degree of muscle relaxation are related to the total dose used. Lidocaine is typically characterized as an agent of intermediate onset and duration. Upper or lower extremity nerve blocks typically require the use of 1% to 2% concentrations with volumes ranging from 15 to 40 ml yielding approximately 1 to 3 hours of surgical anesthesia. The maximum recommended dose of this agent can be increased with the addition of a vasoconstictor such as epinephrine (Table 1.2).

Mepivacaine

Mepivacaine (Carbocaine®) is another commonly used amino-amide local anesthetic characterized by its

Table 1.2 Maximum recommended local anesthetic doses commonly used for peripheral nerve blocks[1]

	Without epinephrine	With epinephrine
2-Chloroprocaine	11 mg/kg (up to 800 mg)	14 mg/kg (up to 1,000 mg)
Lidocaine	5 mg/kg	7 mg/kg
Mepivacaine	5 mg/kg	7–9 mg/kg
Bupivacaine	3 mg/kg	3 mg/kg
Levobupivacaine	3 mg/kg	3 mg/kg
Ropivacaine	3 mg/kg	3 mg/kg

Note: [1]Toxicity data based on intravenous infusion in animals.

intermediate onset and duration. The drug is available in 1%, 1.5%, and 2% concentrations for peripheral nerve blockade. Upper or lower extremity nerve blocks placed using 1.5% or 2% mepivicaine will provide approximately 3 to 6 hours of surgical anesthesia. The dose and duration of mepivacaine can be increased with adjunctive use of a vasoconstrictor, such as epinephrine (Table 1.2). Mepivicaine is usually a good choice for procedures requiring surgical anesthesia without the need for prolonged postoperative analgesia.

Bupivacaine

Bupivacaine (Marcaine®, Sensorcaine®) is characterized as a long-acting amino-amide local anesthetic. Introduced in the 1960s, the drug remains popular today despite the development of newer agents with safer toxicity profiles. Bupivacaine is highly lipid soluble and thus very potent relative to other local anesthetics. The drug's high pKa and strong protein binding affinity correlate with a relatively slower onset when used for peripheral nerve blockade in concentrations between 0.25% and 0.5%. Sensory blockade is usually profound, while motor blockade may be only partial or inadequate for cases where complete muscle relaxation is necessary. Postoperative sensory analgesia is prolonged after bupivacaine use and may last 12 to 24 hours following block placement.

Levobupivacaine

Levobupivacaine (Chirocaine®) is the S-enantiomer of bupivacaine. The drug was developed and

4

marketed in the late 1990s as an alternative to racemic bupivacaine with a safer cardiac toxicity profile. The agent's pharmacologic effect is very similar to bupivacaine, having a relatively slow onset and long duration. The drug is typically used in 0.25% and 0.5% concentrations for peripheral nerve blockade providing 6 to 8 hours of surgical anesthesia.

Ropivacaine

Ropivacaine (Naropin®) is another long-acting amide local anesthetic first marketed in the 1990s. Found to have less cardiac toxicity than bupivacaine in animal models, the drug has grown in popularity as a safer alternative for peripheral nerve blockade where large volumes of anesthetic are required. Ropivacaine is distributed as the isolated S-enantiomer of the drug with a pKa and onset similar to bupivacaine, but slightly less lipid solubility. Sensory blockade when using ropivacaine is typically very strong, with motor blockade being variable, affected by the concentration and total dose of drug administered. Motor blockade may be less than that seen with equal concentrations and volumes of bupivacaine or levobupivacaine (McGlade et al. 1998; Beaulieu et al. 2006). Ropivacaine is available in 0.2%, 0.5%, 0.75%, and 1% concentrations for peripheral nerve blockade. While surgical anesthesia time may be limited to 6 to 8 hours following peripheral nerve blockade, the analgesic effects provided by ropivacaine may extend beyond 12 to 24 hours depending on the concentration used.

Local anesthetic toxicity

Systemic toxicity

Local anesthetic toxicity is a relatively rare, though potentially devastating, complication of regional anesthesia (Table 1.3). Systemic toxicity from local anesthetics can occur as a result of intra-arterial, intravenous, or peripheral tissue injection. Toxic blood and tissue levels will typically manifest as a spectrum of neurological symptoms (ringing in the ears, circumoral numbness and tingling) and signs (muscle twitching, grand mal seizure). If systemic levels of the anesthetic are high enough, respiratory and cardiac involvement with eventual cardiovascular collapse will result. This occurs as local anesthetic molecules avidly bind to voltage-gated sodium channels in cardiac tissue. As it

Table 1.3 Rates of systemic toxic reactions related to local anesthetic use in peripheral nerve blocks by study (without use of ultrasound)

	N	#STR	Rate (frequency/10,000)
1	7,532	15	20
2	21,278	16	7.5
3	9,396	0	0
4	521	1	20

Notes: 1 = Brown et al. 1995; 2 = Auroy et al. 1997; 3 = Giaufre et al. 1996 (pediatric cases only); 4 Borgeat et al. 2001. Revised chart from: Mulroy M (2002) Systemic toxicity and cardio-toxicity from local anesthetics: incidence and preventative measures. Regional Anesthesia and Pain Medicine. 27(6):556–61. #STR = frequency of systemic toxic reactions.

Table 1.4 Relative risk of cardio-toxicity among equivalent doses of amide local anesthetics commonly used for peripheral nerve blockade (greatest to least)

Bupivacaine
Levobupivacaine
Ropivacaine
Mepivacaine
Lidocaine

turns out, bupivacaine does this more readily and with greater intensity than other types of local anesthetics, hence the greater concern for its pro-arrhythmic potential. Ropivacaine and levobupivacaine also share this concern but have a larger therapeutic window: reportedly 40% and 35% respective reductions in cardio-toxic risk as compared with bupivacaine (Table 1.4) (Rathmell et al. 2004).

Recall that signs and symptoms of local anesthetic toxicity can manifest within seconds to hours following injection depending on a number of factors including the amount, site, and route of injection (Tables 1.5 and 1.6). For example, a seizure may occur within seconds of a relatively small intra-arterial injection during an interscalene brachial plexus block, or require many minutes to manifest following placement of an intercostal nerve block with a large volume of concentrated local anesthetic (Table 1.5).

Additional considerations

According to three separate studies, the incidence of systemic toxicity during brachial plexus blockade in

Table 1.5 Factors increasing systemic toxicity of local anesthetics

Local anesthetic choice

Local anesthetic dose

Block location

Decreased protein binding of local anesthetic (low protein states: malnutrition, chronic illness, liver failure, renal failure, etc.)

Acidosis

Peripheral vasoconstriction

Hyperdynamic circulation (this may occur with use of epinephrine)

Table 1.6 Systemic absorption of local anesthetic by site of injection (greatest to least)

Intercostal

Caudal

Paracervical

Epidural

Brachial plexus

Sciatic

adults has been reported from 7.5 to 20 per 10,000 peripheral nerve blocks.

Patient safety is probably improved with some simple safety checks and considerations when bolusing with large volumes of local anesthetic for peripheral nerve blockade: use of less cardio-toxic long-acting agents (ropivacaine and levobupivacaine), incremental aspirations prior to injections, and limiting the total dose of anesthetic administered.

Management of systemic local anesthetic toxicity

In a patient where local anesthetic toxicity is suspected, treatment and supportive care by the anesthesiologist should be undertaken without delay. Emergency airway and resuscitation equipment as well as medications should always be immediately available wherever regional anesthetics are being performed. The airway should be made secure and oxygen provided. If symptoms of central nervous system (CNS) toxicity progress to seizures, medication should be given

to abort the seizure activity. Sodium pentothal 50 to 100 mg or midazolam 2 to 5 mg will often suffice. For cases of complete cardiovascular collapse, advanced cardiac life support (ACLS) protocol should be undertaken. The morbidity and mortality in cases of ventricular fibrillation due to bupivacaine overdose is high, and it is often recommended to consider cardiopulmonary bypass in refractory cases.

Since the late 1990s, increased research has been undertaken regarding the use of lipid emulsion therapy in local anesthetic induced cardio-toxicity. Several laboratory and clinical case reports have now been published reporting successful resuscitative efforts using lipid infusions to counter local anesthetic induced cardio-toxicity. Bolus doses ranging from 1 to 3 ml/kg of 20% lipid emulsion in cases of local anesthetic overdose are typical.

There are theories as to the biologic plausibility of lipid therapy in cases of local anesthetic toxicity. One such theory involves lipid partitioning of the anesthetic away from receptors in tissue ("lipid sink"), thereby alleviating or preventing signs of cardio-toxicity (Weinberg 2008). As more data have become available, it now seems prudent to consider early use of this medication in suspected overdose cases.

Additional considerations

Dosing regimen for lipid emulsion therapy: For suspected local anesthetic toxicity, administer 20% lipid solution 1 ml/kg bolus every 5 minutes up to 3 ml/kg followed by 20% lipid infusion 0.25 ml/kg/min for 3 hours.

Information on lipid emulsion therapy for local anesthetic overdose, including case reports and current research, may be found at LipidRescue™ (www.lipidrescue.org)

Neurotoxicity

Toxicity to nerves during regional anesthetic blockade can occur as a result of local anesthetics themselves or from additives and preservatives within the anesthetic. Local anesthetics do have some neurotoxic effect when applied directly to isolated nerve fibers, though this effect is largely concentration dependent. Lidocaine has specifically been studied for its toxic effect in high concentrations with prolonged exposure to nerve axons (Lambert *et al.* 1994; Kanai *et al.* 2000). This toxic effect is likely multifactorial involving disruption of the nerve's normal homeostatic environment and perhaps changes in intrinsic neural blood blow. Despite findings of some neurotoxic potential, however, the clinical use of local anesthetics in currently recommended concentrations for peripheral nerve blockade is considered safe.

Additives to local anesthetics for peripheral nerve blocks

Additives to local anesthetics for peripheral nerve blockade will have variable effects on block onset time, anesthetic duration, and postoperative analgesia. When deciding on whether or not to use such medications, practitioners should always be aware of the additive drug's pharmacology, effects, and systemic side-effects profile. Integration of this information with the type of local anesthetic to be used, as well as surgical and patient specific factors, may influence the decision to use a particular adjuvant agent.

Epinephrine

Epinephrine is a commonly used additive to local anesthetics when performing peripheral nerve blocks for a number of reasons. Epinephrine has been shown to increase block intensity as well as duration of anesthesia and analgesia with intermediate-acting local anesthetics such as lidocaine and mepivacaine. As a vasoconstrictor with strong alpha-1 effects, epinephrine decreases systemic absorption of the local anesthetic limiting peak plasma levels and prolonging block time. The drug also provides a marker for intravascular injection in dilute concentrations due to its beta-1 effects.

Adjuvant use of epinephrine will have systemic effects, including tachycardia and increased cardiac inotropy, and therefore its use in patients with a significant cardiac history should be carefully considered. The drug should probably be avoided when performing a block to an area receiving diminished or absent anastomotic blood flow. Due to concerns about ischemic neurotoxicity, doses administered in concentrations of 1:400,000 (2.5 mcg/ml) or less may be prudent. Epinephrine administered perineurally decreases extrinsic blood supply when administered in higher concentrations, though there is no evidence this effect is detrimental to humans.

Clonidine

Clonidine is an alpha-2 adrenergic agonist, which has been shown to improve anesthesia and analgesia of peripheral nerve blocks, especially in conjunction with intermediate-acting local anesthetics such as lidocaine and mepivacaine. Use of the drug causes dose-dependent side effects (hypotension, bradycardia, and sedation). By keeping the total dose to <150 mcg, these side effects can be minimized or avoided altogether (Rathmell *et al.* 2004).

Sodium bicarbonate

The addition of sodium bicarbonate to intermediate-acting local anesthetics is often used in an effort to speed onset during peripheral nerve blockade by raising the local anesthetic's pH closer to physiologic pH. In theory, the greater the proportion of the drug in the base (non-ionized) form, the more rapid its passage across the nerve cell membrane to the site where it will have an effect.

In the case of plain mepivacaine or lidocaine, 1 mEq $NaHCO_3$ per 10 ml of local anesthetic is mixed and purported to help speed onset, though this effect is largely unsupported in the literature (Neal *et al.* 2008). There is some evidence of decreased onset time when bicarbonate is added to anesthetics commercially prepared with epinephrine (these preparations tend to be more acidic in nature than plain preparations). The addition of sodium bicarbonate, however, can destabilize local anesthetics. In the case of concentrated preparations of bupivacaine or ropivacaine, the anesthetic will precipitate in solution when mixed with sodium bicarbonate.

Opioids

The use of opioids as an adjuvant for peripheral nerve blocks has largely been shown to be equivocal. One drug, however, has shown some benefit when used in conjunction with local anesthetics for peripheral blocks. Buprenorphine is an opioid agonist-antagonist. Controlling for a systemic effect of the drug, one study has been published showing a prolonged analgesic effect from buprenorphine when administered perineurally with mepivacaine and tetracaine (Candido 2001). Patients administered a dose of 0.3 mg with local anesthetic for axillary brachial plexus block demonstrated an average analgesic duration of 22.3 hours, compared with 12.5 hours for the group receiving local anesthetic with intramuscular (IM) buprenorphine. Nausea, vomiting, and sedation are potential side effects of concern with the use of buprenorphine.

Dexamethasone

The use of the synthetic glucocorticoid dexamethasone as an adjunct to local anesthetics for peripheral nerve blocks is receiving increasing interest. The drug clinically appears to lengthen the sensory, motor, and analgesic time of peripheral nerve blocks when added to both intermediate and longer-acting local anesthetics. The mechanism by which this effect occurs has yet to be determined.

At the time of writing, a number of studies have been published showing a beneficial effect of dexamethasone as an adjunct to local anesthetics in regional anesthesia and pain medicine procedures (see "Suggested reading"). Dexamethasone use in epidural steroid injections is increasingly popular among pain practitioners because of the medication's pharmacologic profile in comparison with other corticosteroids: dexamethasone is non-particulate and void of neurotoxic preservatives (Benzon et al. 2007). It should be noted, however, that current studies assessing the effect of dexamethasone added to plain local anesthetics for peripheral nerve blockade have generally been critiqued as being non-standardized and/or under-powered to achieve statistically significant results (Williams et al. 2009).

Concern over ischemic neurotoxicity has been raised due to the drug's effect, like epinephrine, of decreasing normal nerve tissue blood flow as demonstrated by topical application of 0.4% dexamethasone to the exposed sciatic nerve in rats. As when using epinephrine, it would seem prudent to properly select candidates for adjunctive use of dexamethasone excluding patients at greatest risk for ischemic nerve injury (e.g., poorly controlled diabetes, preexisting nerve injury, or demyelinating disorder).

At the time of publication, there are clinical studies under way looking to further assess the effect of dexamethasone added to local anesthetics for peripheral nerve blocks. Many of these studies are being conducted using 8 mg of dexamethasone or less diluted in a 20- to 40-cc local anesthetic mixture. It has been suggested that additional studies are still needed to further assess the side-effects profile and safety of perineural dexamethasone, in addition to an optimal adjuvant dose, before its use becomes more mainstream (Williams et al. 2009).

Suggested reading

Albright G A. (1979). Cardiac arrest following regional anesthesia with etidocaine or bupivacaine. *Anesthesiology*, **51**:285–7.

Barash P, Cullen B F, Stoelting R K. (2006). *Handbook of Clinical Anesthesia*, 5th edn. Ch 17. Local anesthetics. Lippincott Williams and Wilkins. p. 269.

Beaulieu P, Babin D, Hemmerling T. (2006). The pharmacodynamics of ropivacaine and bupivacaine in combined sciatic and femoral nerve blocks for total knee arthroplasty. *Anesth Analg*, **103**:768–74.

Benzon H T, Chew T L, McCarthy R J, Benzon H A, Walega D R. (2007).Comparison of the particle sizes of different steroids and the effect of dilution: a review of the relative neurotoxicities of the steroids. *Anesthesiology*, **106**(2):331–8.

Bigat Z, Boztug N, Hadimioglu N, et al. (2006). Does dexamethasone improve the quality of intravenous regional anesthesia and analgesia? A randomized, controlled clinical study. *Anesth Analg*, **102**(2):605–9.

Candido K. (2001). Buprenorphine added to the local anesthetic for brachial plexus block to provide postoperative analgesia in outpatients. *Reg Anesth Pain Med*, **26**(4):352–6.

Drager C, Benziger D, Gao F, Berde C B. (1998). Prolonged intercostal nerve blockade in sheep using controlled-release of bupivacaine and dexamethasone from polymer microspheres. *Anesthesiology*, **89**(4):969–79.

Estebe J P, LeCorre P, Clement R, et al. (2003). Effect of dexamethasone on motor brachial plexus block with bupivacaine and with bupivacaine loaded microspheres in a sheep model. *Eur J Anaesthesiol*, **20**(4):305–10.

Fernández-Guisasola J, Andueza A, Burgos E, et al. (2008). A comparison of 0.5% ropivacaine and 1% mepivacaine for sciatic nerve block in the popliteal fossa. *Acta Anaesthesiol Scand*, **45**(8):967–70.

Fujii Y, Tanaka H, Toyooka H. (1997). The effects of dexamethasone on antiemetics in female patients undergoing gynecologic surgery. *Anesth Analg*, **85**(4):913–17.

Henzi I, Walder B, Tramer, M R. (2000). Dexamethasone for prevention of postoperative nausea and vomiting: a quantitative systematic review. *Anesth Analg*, **90**(1):186–94.

Kanai Y, Katsuki H, Takasaki M. (2000). Lidocaine disrupts axonal membrane of rat sciatic nerve in vitro. *Anesth Analg*, **91**(4):944–8.

Kopacz D J, Lacouture P G, Wu D, *et al.* (2003). The dose response and effects of dexamethasone on bupivacaine microcapsules for intercostal blockade (T9–T11) in healthy volunteers. *Anesth Analg*, **96**(2):576–82.

Lambert L, Lambert D, Strichartz G. (1994). Irreversible conduction block in isolated nerve by high concentrations of local anesthetics. *Anesthesiology*, **80**(5):1082–93.

Ludot H, Tharin J Y, Belouadah M, Mazoit J X, Malinovsky J M. (2008). Successful resuscitation after ropivacaine and lidocaine-induced ventricular arrhythmia following posterior lumbar plexus block in a child. *Anesth Analg*, **106**(5):1572–3.

McGlade D P, Kalpokas M V, Mooney P H, *et al.* (1998). A comparison of 0.5% ropivacaine and 0.5% bupivacaine for axillary brachial plexus anesthesia. *Anaesth Intensive Care*, **26**(5):515–20.

Movafegh A, Razazian M, Hajimaohamadi F, Meysamie A. (2006). Dexamethasone added to lidocaine prolongs axillary brachial plexus blockade. *Anesth Analg*, **102**(1):263–7.

Mulroy M. (2002). Systemic toxicity and cardiotoxicity from local anesthetics: incidence and preventative measures. *Reg Anesth Pain Med*, **27**(6):556–61.

Neal J M, Gerancher J C, Hebl J R, *et al.* (2009). Upper extremity regional anesthesia: essentials of our current understanding. *Reg Anesth Pain Med*, **34**(2):134–70.

Rathmell J P, Neal J M, Viscomi C M. (2004). *Regional Anesthesia: The Requisites in Anesthesiology*. Chapter 2. Pharmacology of local anesthetics. St Louis: Elsevier Mosby Publishing.

Shishido H, Shinichi K, Heckman H, Myers R. (2002). Dexamethasone decreases blood flow in normal nerves and dorsal root ganglia. *Spine*, **27**(6):581–6.

Shrestha B R, Maharjan S K, Tabedar S. (2003). Supraclavicular brachial plexus block with and without dexamethasone – a comparative study. *Kathmandu Univ Med J*, **1**(3):158–60.

Shrestha B R, Maharjan S K, Shrestha S, *et al.* (2007). Comparative study between tramadol and dexamethasone as an admixture to bupivicaine in supraclavicular brachial plexus block. *J Nepal Med Assoc*, **46**(168):158–64.

Thomas S, Beevi S. (2006). Epidural dexamethasone reduces postoperative pain and analgesic requirements *Can J Anesth*, **53**(9):899–905.

Tzeng J I, Wang J J, Ho S T, *et al.* (2000). Dexamethasone for prophylaxis of nausea and vomiting after epidural morphine for post-Caesarean section analgesia: comparison of droperidol and saline. *Br J Anesth*, **85**(6):865–8.

Wang J J, Ho S T, Wong C S, *et al.* (2001). Dexamethasone prophylaxis of nausea and vomiting after epidural morphine for post-Cesarean analgesia. *Can J Anesth*, **48**(2):185–90.

Wang J J, Lee S C, Liu Y C, Ho C M. (2000). The use of dexamethasone for preventing postoperative nausea and vomiting in females undergoing thyroidectomy: a dose ranging study. *Anesth Analg*, **91**(6):1404–7.

Weinberg, G L. (2008). Lipid infusion therapy: translation to clinical practice. *Anesth Analg*, **106**(5):1340–2.

Weinberg G L. (2010). http://lipidrescue.org. University of Illinois, College of Medicine, Chicago.

Weinberg G L, VadeBoncouer T, Ramaraju G A, Garcia-Amaro M F, Cwik M J. (1998). Pretreatment or resuscitation with a lipid infusion shifts the dose-response to bupivacaine-induced asystole in rats. *Anesthesiology*, **88**(4):1071–5.

Weinberg G L, Ripper R, Feinstein D L, Hoffman W. (2003). Lipid emulsion infusion rescue in dogs from bupivacaine-induced cardiac toxicity. *Reg Anesth Pain Med*, **28**:198–202.

Weinberg G L, Ripper R, Murphy P, *et al.* (2006). Lipid infusion accelerates removal of bupivacaine and recovery from bupivacaine toxicity in the isolated rat heart. *Reg Anesth Pain Med*, **31**(4):296–303.

Williams B A, Murinson B B, Grable B R, Orebaugh S L. (2009). Future considerations for pharmacologic adjuvants in single-injection peripheral nerve blocks for patients with diabetes mellitus. *Reg Anesth Pain Med*, **34**(5):445–57.

Chapter 2

Introduction to ultrasound

Introduction

The use of ultrasound guidance in regional anesthesia is an ever-evolving field with changing technology. This chapter provides a brief overview of the physics involved in two-dimensional ultrasound image generation, ultrasound probe types and machine control features, basic tissue imaging characteristics, and imaging artifacts commonly seen during performance of a regional ultrasound-guided procedure.

Image generation

Ultrasound waves are generated by piezoelectric crystals in the handheld probe. Piezoelectric crystals generate an electrical current when a mechanical stress is applied to them. Therefore, the generation of an electrical current when a mechanical stress is applied is called the *piezoelectric effect.* The reverse can also occur via the *converse piezoelectric effect*, so that an electrical current applied to piezoelectric crystals can induce mechanical stress and deformation. Ultrasound waves are generated via the converse piezoelectric effect. Application of an electrical current to the piezoelectric crystals in the handheld probe causes cyclical deformation of the crystals, which leads to generation of ultrasound waves.

The ultrasound probe acts as both a transmitter and receiver (Figure 2.1). The probe cycles between generating ultrasound waves 1% of the time and "listening" for the return of ultrasound waves or "echoes" 99% of the time. Using the piezoelectric effect, the piezoelectric crystals in the handheld probe convert the mechanical energy of the returning echoes into an electrical current, which is processed by the machine to produce a two-dimensional grayscale image that is seen on the screen. The image on the screen can range from black to white. The greater the

energy from the returning echoes from an area, the whiter the image will appear.

- **Hyperechoic** areas have a great amount of energy from returning echoes and are seen as white.
- **Hypoechoic** areas have less energy from returning echoes and are seen as gray.
- **Anechoic** areas without returning echoes are seen as black (Table 2.1).

Generation of images requires reflection of ultrasound waves back to the probe to be processed, this reflection occurs at the boundary or interface of different types of tissue. *Acoustic impedance* is the resistance to the passage of ultrasound waves, the greater the acoustic impedance, the more resistant that tissue is to the passage of ultrasound waves. The greatest reflection of echoes back to the probe comes from interfaces of tissues with the greatest difference in acoustic impedance (Table 2.2). From Table 2.2 we can see that there is a large difference between the acoustic impedance of air and soft tissue, which is why any interface between air and soft tissue will give a hyperechoic image. There is also a large difference between the acoustic impedance of bone and soft tissue, therefore, bone and soft tissue interfaces will also give a hyperechoic image. The difference in acoustic impedance between various types of soft tissue, such as blood, muscle, and fat, are very small and result in hypoechoic images.

Other imaging technologies used in medicine, such as X-rays or computed tomography (CT) scans can show density directly. However, ultrasound imaging is based on the differences in acoustic impedance at tissue interfaces. A hyperechoic image on ultrasound should not be interpreted as more dense and a hypoechoic image as less dense. Recall that both bone and air bubbles can give hyperechoic images, yet they have very different densities.

Table 2.1 Appearance of anechoic, hypoechoic, and hyperechoic areas

Anechoic	Black
Hypoechoic	Gray
Hyperechoic	White

Table 2.2 Acoustic impedance of various human tissues

Body tissue	Acoustic impedance (10^6 Rayls)
Air	0.0004
Fat	1.35
Blood	1.70
Muscle	1.75
Bone	7.8

Table 2.3

Medium	Ultrasound Speed (m/sec) (acoustic velocity)
Air	300
Lung	500
Fat	1,450
Soft Tissue	1,540
Bone	4,000

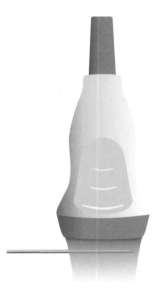

Figure 2.2 Needle is perpendicular to the path of the ultrasound beam.

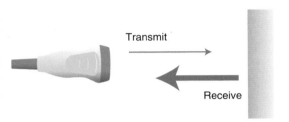

Figure 2.1 Ultrasound probes act as both transmitters and receivers.

Ultrasound waves and tissue interaction

The speed of ultrasound waves through biological tissue is based on the density of the tissue, and not the frequency of the ultrasound wave. Table 2.3 shows the speed of ultrasound in various tissues, the greater the tissue density, the faster the ultrasound waves will travel. The image processor in the ultrasound machine assumes that the ultrasound waves are traveling through soft tissue at a velocity of 1,540 m/sec. This assumption leads to image artifacts, which will be discussed later in the chapter. Three things can happen to ultrasound waves as they travel through tissue – *reflection, attenuation, and refraction* – each will be discussed in detail below (Figure 2.7).

Reflection

The generation of ultrasound images is dependent on the energy of the echoes that return to the probe.

The amount of reflection of ultrasound waves is dependent on the difference in acoustic impedance at the interface between different tissues. *Acoustic impedance* is the resistance of a material to the passage of ultrasound waves. The greater the difference in acoustic impedance at tissue interfaces, the greater the percentage of ultrasound waves that is reflected back to the probe to be processed into an image.

The angle of incidence is an important factor in determining the amount of reflection that occurs. The more perpendicular an object is to the path of the ultrasound waves, the more reflection that will occur and the more parallel an object is to the path of the ultrasound waves, the less reflection that will occur (Figures 2.2 and 2.3). Therefore, in order to better visualize the block needle, the needle should be inserted as perpendicular to the path of the ultrasound waves as the block technique allows. Blocks of deeper nerves require the needle to be inserted more parallel to the ultrasound waves, which makes visualization of the needle difficult. **A needle inserted at a shallow angle to the probe will be easier to visualize than one inserted at a steep angle to the probe.**

There are two types of reflectors – specular and scattering.

1. A **specular reflector** is a large and smooth reflector such as a block needle, diaphragm, or the

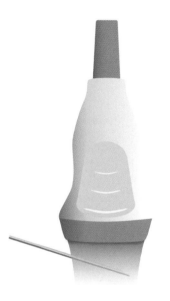

Figure 2.3 Needle is not as perpendicular to the ultrasound beam as in Figure 2.3, and will be more difficult to image.

walls of large vessels. The ultrasound waves are reflected in one direction back to the ultrasound probe (Figure 2.4). In specular reflection, the angle of incidence equals the angle of return. In order for specular reflection to occur, the wavelength of the ultrasound wave must be shorter than the size of the object. High-frequency probes have shorter wavelengths thus allowing for imaging of smaller objects through specular reflection. Specular reflection allows a greater percentage of ultrasound waves to return directly to the probe to be processed into an image. Due to this greater return of waves, specular reflectors generally give a hyperechoic image.

2. A **scattering reflector** is an object with an irregular surface that, as the name implies, "scatters" the ultrasound wave in multiple directions and at varying angles towards and away from the probe (Figure 2.4). Scattering occurs when the ultrasound wave encounters small objects and objects that are not smooth, or when the wavelength of the ultrasound wave is longer than

Specular reflector    Diffuse reflector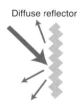

Figure 2.4 Specular reflection vs. scattering reflection.

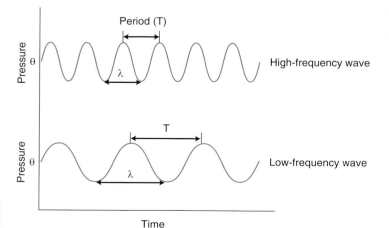

Figure 2.5 High-frequency probes produce shorter wavelength waves, and low-frequency probes produce longer wavelength waves.

the size of the object. Low-frequency probes have longer wavelengths. Due to scattering, fewer waves return to the probe to be processed into an image.

The equation $c = \lambda \times f$ can be used to represent an ultrasound wave in the human body. Where λ represents wavelength, f represents frequency, and c is the speed of sound through human tissue, which the processor assumes to be 1,540 m/sec. Based on this equation the higher the frequency of a wave, the shorter the wavelength, and the lower the frequency of a wave, the longer the wavelength. Therefore, high-frequency probes produce shorter wavelength ultrasound waves, and low-frequency probes produce longer wavelength ultrasound waves (Figure 2.5). Shorter wavelength ultrasound waves allow imaging of smaller objects through specular reflection rather than scattering reflection.

Attenuation

Attenuation is the loss of mechanical energy of ultrasound waves as they travel through tissue. About 75% of attenuation is caused by conversion to heat, which is called *absorption*. The greater the *attenuation coefficient* of a tissue, the greater the loss of energy of ultrasound waves as they travel through the tissue (Table 2.4).

Attenuation of ultrasound waves is dependent on three factors (1) the attenuation coefficient of the tissue, (2) the distance traveled, and (3) the frequency of the ultrasound waves. Attenuation is inversely related to frequency; the higher the frequency of the ultrasound wave, the greater the attenuation. Therefore, high-frequency probes have less tissue penetration due to greater attenuation, which makes imaging of deeper structures difficult with high-frequency probes.

Refraction

When the acoustic impedance between tissue interfaces is small, the ultrasound wave's direction is changed slightly at the tissue interface, rather than being reflected directly back to the probe at the interface (Figures 2.6 and 2.7). This is analogous to the bent appearance of a fork in water, which is caused by refraction of light waves at the air/water interface. Refracted waves may not return to the probe in order to be processed into an image. Therefore, refraction may contribute to image degradation.

Resolution

Resolution, the ability to distinguish two close objects as separate, is very important in ultrasound-guided

Table 2.4 Attenuation coefficient of different tissue at a frequency of 1 MHz

Body tissue	Attenuation coefficient (dB/cm at 1 MHz)
Water	0.002
Blood	0.18
Fat	0.65
Muscle	1.5–3.5
Bone	5.0

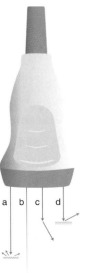

Figure 2.7 (a) Scattering reflection, (b) attenuation, (c) refraction, (d) specular reflection.

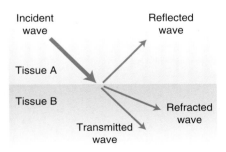

Figure 2.6 Refraction vs. reflection.

regional anesthesia. There are two types of resolution – axial and lateral.

Axial resolution

Axial resolution is the ability to distinguish two objects that lie in a plane parallel to the direction of the ultrasound beam. Axial resolution is equal to half of the pulse length. Higher frequency probes have shorter pulse lengths, which allows for better axial resolution (Figure 2.9a and b).

The ultrasound probe emits ultrasound waves in pulses, not continuously (Figure 2.8). These pulses of ultrasound waves are emitted intermittently as the probe has to wait and listen for the returning echoes.

- **Pulse**: a few sound waves of similar frequency.
- **Pulse length**: the distance a pulse travels.
- **Pulse repetition frequency:** the rate at which pulses are emitted per unit of time.

Lateral resolution

Lateral resolution is the ability to distinguish two objects that lie in a plane perpendicular to the direction of the ultrasound beam (Figure 2.10). Lateral resolution is related to the ultrasound beam width. The more narrow (focused) the ultrasound beam width, the greater the lateral resolution. High-frequency probes have narrower beam widths, which allows for better lateral resolution. Poor lateral resolution means that two objects lying side by side may be seen as one object. The position of the narrowest part of the beam can be adjusted by changing the focal zone.

The *near field* is the non-diverging part of the ultrasound beam and as the name suggests is close to the ultrasound probe. The *far field* is the diverging portion of the ultrasound beam that is farther away from the transducer. The *focal zone* is the narrowest

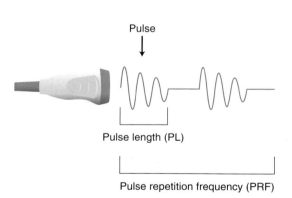

Figure 2.8 The ultrasound probe emits ultrasound waves in pulses, not continuously.

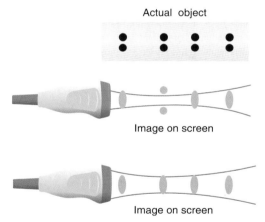

Figure 2.10 Lateral resolution.

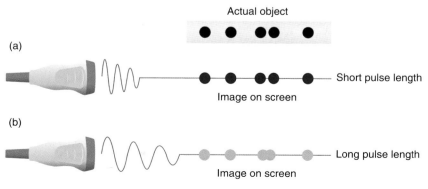

Figure 2.9 (a) High-frequency probe; (b) low-frequency probe.

part of the beam and the area of the best lateral resolution (Figure 2.11). High-frequency probes have narrower beam widths and better near-field resolution. The focal zone can be adjusted manually on some ultrasound machines (Figure 2.12).

Key points

High-frequency probes have better axial and lateral resolution, but greater tissue attenuation, which decreases tissue penetration. Therefore, high-frequency probes are better for imaging small and superficial structures.

Low-frequency probes have greater tissue penetration but poorer axial and lateral resolution. Low-frequency probes are better for imaging deep structures of larger size.

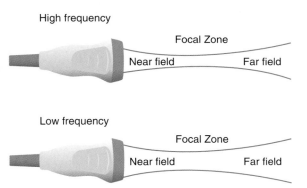

Figure 2.11 High-frequency probes have narrower focal zones and better near-field resolution.

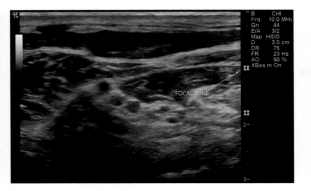

Figure 2.12 The area between the hour glass figures represents the focal zone and can be adjusted manually on some ultrasound machines.

Ultrasound equipment
Introduction
The use of ultrasound guidance in regional anesthesia is an ever-evolving technology. A number of different portable ultrasound machines are available making their use in anesthesiology more practical than ever. Due to the variety of machines and the constantly evolving technology it would be impossible to discuss each individual machine. However, a discussion of some of the current technology and controls common to most machines is useful for the regional anesthesiologist.

Ultrasound transducers
Ultrasound transducers, or probes, can be categorized based on their frequency range, low frequency vs. high frequency, and the shape of the probe, curved vs. linear. Linear array probes are high-frequency probes. High-frequency probes have less tissue penetration but good near-field image resolution. Curved array probes are low-frequency probes. Low-frequency probes have greater tissue penetration; however, resolution is compromised.

The *footprint* of a probe refers to the physical size of the part of the ultrasound probe that contacts the patient. The *field of view* is the width of the image that is seen on the screen. The field of view of a linear array probe is constant and is the size of the probe's footprint (Figure 2.13).

The field of view of a curved array probe (measured in degrees) diverges as it exits the probe and is not constant (Figure 2.14). The divergence of ultrasound waves gives curved array probes a much wider

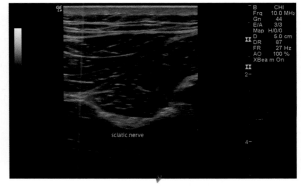

Figure 2.13 Subgluteal sciatic nerve block with a high-frequency linear array probe.

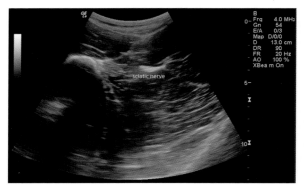

Figure 2.14 Subgluteal sciatic nerve block with a low-frequency curved array probe.

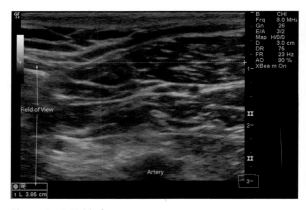

Figure 2.15 Field of view.

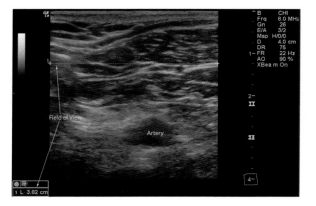

Figure 2.16 Field of view.

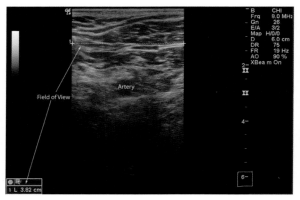

Figure 2.17 Field of view is constant from a depth of 3 cm to 6 cm at 3.85 cm.

field of view. However, divergence can cause some image distortion. One advantage of divergence is that a needle inserted in plane can be in the ultrasound beam and visualized prior to the needle being physically under the probe. This characteristic may allow visualization of the needle earlier than with a linear array probe. This advantage must be balanced against the lower resolution of low-frequency curved array probes and the image distortion caused by divergence of ultrasound beams.

Ultrasound machine controls

Depth

The depth of tissue imaged can be adjusted on the machine and relates to the type of probe being used. Low-frequency probes will be able to image deeper tissue depths than high-frequency probes.

With a linear array probe, as the depth is increased, the image on the screen will appear narrower and structures will appear smaller, but the

width of the field of view is relatively constant. Notice that the field of view is constant from 3 cm to 6 cm (Figures 2.15–2.17), but at 2 cm it has decreased (Figure 2.18).

Frequency

Variable-frequency probes allow changes in frequency within a narrow range. An 8 to 13 MHz probe allows selection of frequency between 8 and 13 MHz. The lower frequencies are used for deeper structures and the higher frequencies are used for more superficial structures. Select a frequency that balances penetration and resolution.

Gain

Ultrasound probes transmit ultrasound waves 1% of the time and spend the remaining 99% of the time listening for the returning echoes. Increasing the gain,

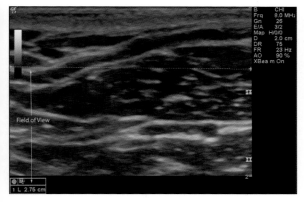

Figure 2.18 Field of view at a depth of 2 cm has decreased to 2.75 cm.

increases signal amplification of the returning ultrasound waves, in this way the gain function can be used to compensate for loss of energy due to tissue attenuation (Figure 2.19). Returning ultrasound waves are referred to as "signal" while background artifact is referred to as "noise". Increasing the gain, increases the signal-to-noise ratio. However, if the gain is increased too much, the screen will have a "white out" appearance and all useful information is lost.

Time gain compensation (TGC) allows selective control of gain at different depths (Figure 2.19). Ultrasound waves returning from deeper structures have undergone greater attenuation. To compensate for the loss of signal intensity, TGC allows for stepwise increase in gain to compensate for greater attenuation of ultrasound waves returning from deeper structures. Time gain compensation controls should be moved to the right in a stepwise fashion to "amplify" the returning signal from the deeper structures.

Color-flow Doppler

Color-flow Doppler allows for detection of flow within vascular structures. Moving objects, such as red blood cells (RBCs), affect returning ultrasound waves differently than stationary objects. Color-flow Doppler can differentiate between RBCs moving away from the probe and RBCs moving towards the probe. Red blood cells moving towards the probe will return ultrasound waves at a higher frequency and are displayed as red, RBCs moving away from the probe will return ultrasound waves at a lower frequency and are displayed as blue (Figures 2.21 and 2.22). By changing the angle of the probe to the skin, the flow can be seen

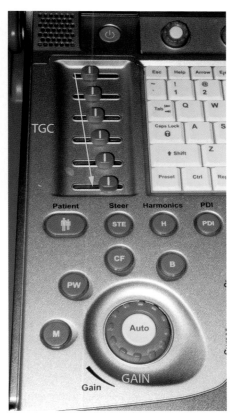

Figure 2.19 Gain and time gain compensation (TGC).

as either red or blue. When the probe is perpendicular to the skin, detection of flow is difficult (Figure 2.20). Therefore, the color displayed is not a reliable indicator of arterial vs. venous flow. The more parallel the probe is to the direction of flow, the easier it is for the ultrasound machine to detect flow. With the ultrasound machine in the color-flow Doppler mode, increasing the gain increases the sensitivity to flow signals. Sometimes very high sensitivity to flow signals is needed when using color-flow Doppler to detect blood flow in smaller vessels.

Pulse-wave Doppler

Pulse-wave Doppler provides flow data from a small area along the ultrasound beam (Figures 2.23 and 2.24). The area to be sampled can be selected by the operator. Once pulse-wave Doppler is selected, the image is frozen and the operator selects the area to be sampled. The pulse-wave information is displayed graphically at the bottom of the screen as well as heard.

17

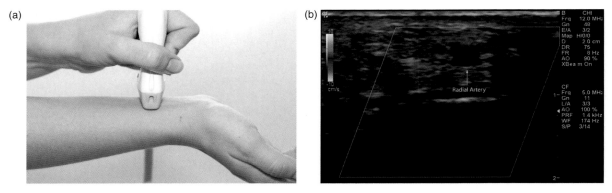

Figure 2.20b Flow not detected with the probe perpendicular to the direction of flow.

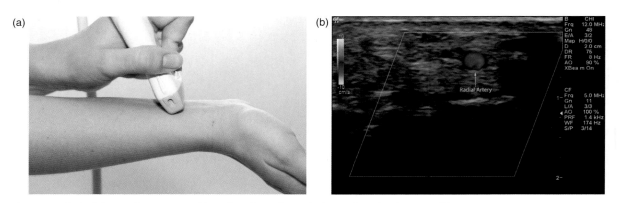

Figure 2.21b Radial artery flow is seen as blue when the probe is tilted away from the direction of flow.

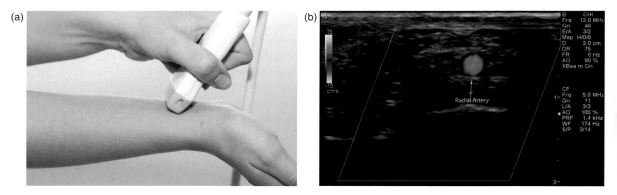

Figure 2.22b Radial artery flow is seen as red when the probe is tilted towards the direction of flow.

Tissue appearance under ultrasound

Computer generated two-dimensional images seen on the ultrasound machine range from white to black (Table 2.5). Strongly reflected waves, such as those from specular reflectors and those from boundaries of tissues with great differences in acoustic impedance (bone/soft tissue), will have a white or **hyperechoic** appearance. Examples of hyperechoic appearance would be bone, diaphragm, or a block needle.

Ultrasound waves from scattering reflectors or those returning from deeper regions that have undergone extensive attenuation have a gray or **hypoechoic**

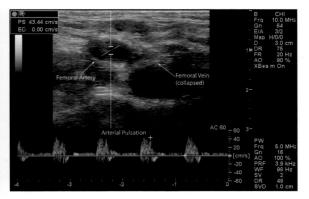

Figure 2.23 Pulse-wave Doppler showing arterial flow in the femoral artery.

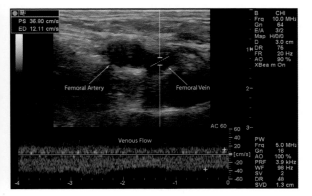

Figure 2.24 Pulse-wave Doppler showing venous flow in the femoral vein.

Table 2.5 Ultrasound image of various tissues for regional anesthesia

Tissue	Ultrasound image for regional anesthesia
Arteries	Anechoic/hypoechoic, pulsatile, non-compressible (Figure 2.25)
Veins	Anechoic/hypoechoic, non-pulsatile, compressible (Figure 2.26)
Fat	Hypoechoic, compressible (Figure 2.27)
Muscles	Heterogeneous (mixture of hyperechoic lines within a hypoechoic tissue background) (Figure 2.27)
Tendons/ fascia	Hyperechoic (Figure 2.28)
Bone	Very hyperechoic with acoustic shadowing behind (Figure 2.29)
Nerves	Hyperechoic below the clavicle/ hypoechoic above the clavicle (Figures 2.28–2.31)
Air bubbles	Hyperechoic (Figure 2.31)
Pleura	Hyperechoic line
Local anesthetic	Hypoechoic, expanding hypoechoic region (Figure 2.32)

appearance. Examples of hypoechoeic appearance would be soft tissue, such as muscle, solid organs, and fat.

When waves are not reflected and travel unimpeded, the structure will have a black, or **anechoeic** appearance. Large blood vessels have an anaechoic appearance because the ultrasound waves travel through blood, which is relatively homogenous in its acoustic impedance, without being reflected. Also, any structure behind a highly reflective surface will have an anaechoic appearance. A highly reflective surface, such as bone, does not allow any ultrasound waves to penetrate. Therefore, structures behind highly reflective surfaces cannot be visualized (Table 2.5).

- *Arteries/veins:* the homogenous nature of blood allows for passage of ultrasound waves without much reflection, which leads to the anechoic appearance of large arteries and veins. Smaller arteries and veins are seen as hypoechoic. Veins are compressible due to their thin walls and low pressure. Arteries are pulsatile, with larger arteries being non-compressible (Figures 2.25 and 2.26).
- *Fat:* hypoechoic background with hyperechoic lines. Fat is compressible whereas muscle and nerves are not compressible (Figure 2.27).
- *Muscle:* hypoechoic background with hyperechoic lines. Muscle is not compressible and may be surrounded by a bright hyperechoic line representing fascia (Figure 2.27).
- *Tendons:* hyperechoic. Nerves scanned in the longitudinal plane may be confused with tendons. Tendons should become larger as they attach to muscles. Tracing the course of a tendon should lead to a muscle, whereas nerves should stay consistent in shape and size.
- *Fascia:* bright hyperechoic line (Figure 2.28).
- *Bone:* bone is very hyperechoic bright white lines. Bone will have an anechoic shadow behind due to the inability of ultrasound waves to penetrate bone (Figure 2.29).

19

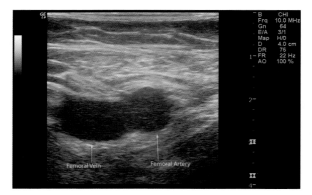

Figure 2.25 Femoral artery and vein.

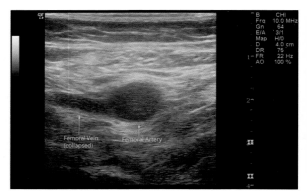

Figure 2.26 With slight pressure of the probe the femoral vein is collapsed.

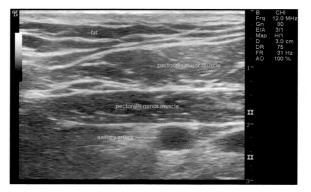

Figure 2.27 Muscle and fat in the infraclavicular region.

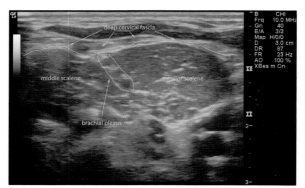

Figure 2.28 Interscalene region with the deep cervical fascia as a hyperechoic line. Trunks of the brachial plexus seen as round hypoechoic structures.

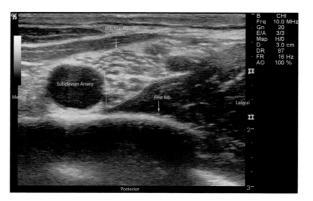

Figure 2.29 The supraclavicular region. The first rib appears as a bright hyperechoic line. Ultrasound is unable to visualize structures deep to the first rib, which creates an acoustic shadowing artifact behind bone.

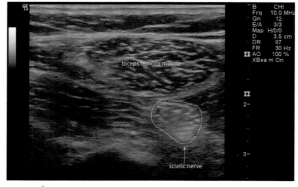

Figure 2.30 Sciatic nerve as a hyperechoic round sturcture with internal hypoechoic structures.

- *Nerves:* nerves may appear as hyperechoic or hypoechoic. Nerves above the clavicle appear hypoechoic (Figures 2.28, 2.29, 2.32) and below the clavicle appear hyperechoic (Figures 2.30 and 2.31). Neural tissue itself is hypoechoic. It is the connective tissue that surrounds nerves that give some nerves their hyperechoic appearance. Large nerves, such as the sciatic

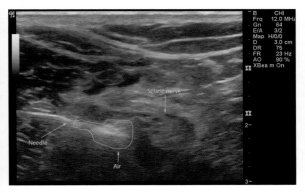

Figure 2.31 Air artifact during a sciatic nerve block in the popliteal fossa.

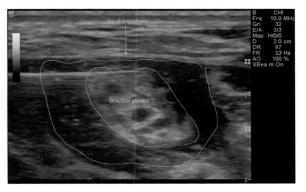

Figure 2.32 Hypoechoic area surrounding the trunks of the brachial plexus in the interscalene region.

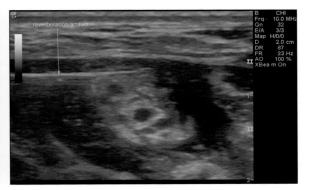

Figure 2.33 Reverberation artifact with a 22-gage needle during an interscalene brachial plexus block.

nerve, may show internal fascicular structure in the transverse view. Some nerves can appear as hyperechoic or hypoechoic depending on the angle of the ultrasound beam to the nerve, this property is called *anisotropy*. The sciatic nerve displays a great deal of anisotropy. Slight angle changes of the probe will aid in bringing the sciatic nerve into view.

- *Air bubbles:* air bubbles injected into tissue have a highly hyperechoic appearance. The large difference in the attenuation coefficient of air and soft tissue causes a large amount of reflection of ultrasound waves, which is interpreted as a hyperechoic image. Hyperechoic areas caused by air bubbles can compromise imaging. It is very important to remove all air bubbles from syringes of local anesthetic (Figure 2.31).

- *Local anesthetic*: injection of local anesthetic is seen as an expanding hypoechoic region (Figure 2.32).
- *Pleura*: hyperechoic. Not as attenuating as bone, so areas distal to pleura may be hypoechoic compared to areas distal to bone, which are anechoic. May be seen during a supraclavicular block.

Artifacts
Reverberation artifact
The processing unit in the ultrasound machine assumes echoes return directly to the processor from the point of reflection. Depth is calculated as $D = V \times T$, where V is the speed of sound in biological tissue and assumed to be 1,540 m/sec, and T is time. In a reverberation artifact, the ultrasound waves bounce back and forth between two interfaces (in this case the lumen of the needle) before returning to the transducer. Since velocity is assumed to be constant at 1,540 m/sec by the processor, the delay in the return of these echoes is interpreted as another structure deep to the needle and hence the multiple hyperechoic lines beneath the block needle (Figure 2.33).

Mirror artifact
A mirror artifact is a type of reverberation artifact. The ultrasound waves bounce back and forth in the lumen of a large vessel (subclavian artery). The delay in time of returning waves to the processor is interpreted by the machine as another vessel distal to the actual vessel (Figure 2.34).

21

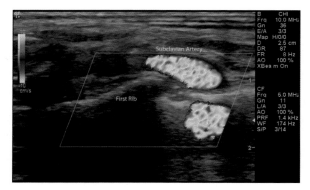

Figure 2.34 Mirror artifact of the subclavian artery during a supraclavicular nerve block.

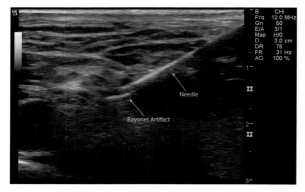

Figure 2.35 Bayonet artifact with a Touhy needle during a supraclavicular catheter placement.

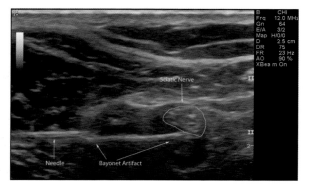

Figure 2.36 Bayonet artifact with a 21-gage needle during a sciatic nerve block in the popliteal fossa.

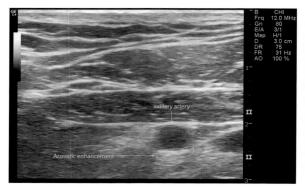

Figure 2.37 Acoustic enhancement seen distal to the axillary artery during an infraclavicular block. May be confused with the posterior cord of the brachial plexus.

Bayonet artifact

The processor assumes that the ultrasound waves travel at 1,540 m/sec through biological tissue. However, we know that there are slight differences in the speed of ultrasound through different biological tissues. The delay in return of echoes from tissue that has slower transmission speed, coupled with the processor's assumption that the speed of ultrasound is constant, causes the processor to interpret these later returning echoes from the tip of the needle traveling in tissue with slower transmission speed as being from a deeper structure and thus giving a bayoneted appearance. If the tip is traveling through tissue that has faster transmission speed, then the bayoneted portion will appear closer to the transducer (Figures 2.35 and 2.36).

Acoustic enhancement artifact

Acoustic enhancement artifacts occur distal to areas where ultrasound waves have traveled through a medium that is a weak attenuator, such as a large blood vessel. Enhancement artifacts are typically seen distal to the femoral and the axillary artery (Figures 2.37 and 2.38).

Absent blood flow

The color-flow Doppler may not detect flow when the ultrasound probe is perpendicular to the direction of flow. A small tilt of the probe away from the perpendicular should visualize the flow (Figures 2.20–2.22). Alternatively, for deep vascular structures, signal may be lost due to attenuation. Increasing gain, while in Doppler color-flow mode, will increase the intensity of the returning signals, which may detect flow that was not previously detected.

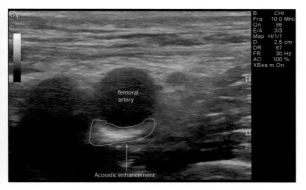

Figure 2.38 Acoustic enhancement artifact seen distal to the femoral artery during a femoral nerve block.

Acoustic shadowing

Tissues with high attenuation coefficients, such as bone, do not allow passage of ultrasound waves. Therefore any structure lying behind tissue with a high attenuation coefficient cannot be imaged and will be seen as an anechoic region. (Figure 2.29)

Suggested reading

Bianchi S, Martinoli C. (2007). *Ultrasound of the Musculoskeletal System.* Springer.

McGahan J P, Goldberg B B. (2007). *Diagnostic Ultrasound,* Volume 1. Informa Healthcare USA.

Sites B D, Brull R, Chan V W S, *et al.* (2007). Artifacts and pitfall errors associated with ultrasound-guided regional anesthesia. Part I: Understanding the basic principles of ultrasound physics and machine operations. *Reg Anesth,* **32**(5):412–18.

Sites B D, Brull R, Chan V W S, *et al.* (2007). Artifacts and pitfall errors associated with ultrasound-guided regional anesthesia. Part II: A pictoral approach to understanding and avoidance. *Reg Anesth,* **32**(5):419–33.

Sprawls P. (1993). *Physical Principle of Medical Imaging,* 2nd edn. Medical Physics Publishing.

Chapter 3

Application of ultrasound in regional anesthesia

Probe preparation

When performing an ultrasound-guided regional anesthesia procedure, ultrasound transducers should be covered with a sterile dressing to protect the transducer and the patient from contamination. Either a sterile transparent dressing (Tegaderm™; 3M Health Care, St Paul, MN, USA) or an ultrasound transducer sheath can be used (Figures 3.1 and 3.2).

Ultrasound transducers should be cleaned with a non-alcohol based cleaner. Alcohol-based cleaners can cause the rubber diaphragm of the probe to dry and crack.

Sterile conduction gel is used to cover the tip of the transducer. As discussed in Chapter 2, Introduction to ultrasound, the speed of ultrasound waves in air is very slow. Any pockets of air between the transducer and the patient will lead to very poor image acquisition and artifacts (Figure 3.3). Conduction gel eliminates any pockets of air that exist between the transducer and the patient. A small amount of gel is sufficient, as too much gel will make handling the transducer difficult. If a transducer sheath is used, conduction gel should also be placed in the sheath to eliminate any pockets of air between the probe and the sheath (Figure 3.2).

Physician and patient positioning

Maintaining a steady ultrasound image on the screen is very important for performing successful ultrasound-guided peripheral nerve blocks. While proper patient position and probe handling are important for maintaining a steady image, physician positioning during the procedure is often overlooked.

When starting a scanning procedure, the patient should be positioned at a height that allows the operator to comfortably stand straight, without having to hunch over excessively. Uncomfortable physician posture can lead to back pain and fatigue during the procedure. The physician's body should be braced

against the bed with a portion of the scanning forearm, wrist, or hand always resting on the patient to provide a stable platform (Figure 3.4). Failure to stabilize the probe with a portion of arm on the patient can lead to shaking of the probe and image distortion as the operator's arm and shoulder begin to fatigue (Figure 3.5). Proper body mechanics are even more important for the novice, as the time required to perform peripheral nerve blocks will be longer for a beginner.

Scanning
Orientation marker

Ultrasound probes have a mark that corresponds to a mark on the ultrasound machine's screen (Figure 3.6a and b). By convention, this orientation marker is placed to the right of the patient when the probe is in a transverse plane to the patient's body, and placed cephalad when the probe is in a longitudinal plane to the patient's body.

Transverse scan

During a transverse scan, the ultrasound probe is placed in a perpendicular plane to the target being imaged (Figure 3.7a and b). The image on the screen is a cross-sectional view of the nerve or blood vessel. During a transverse scan, nerves and vessels appear round. The terms transverse, short axis, and out-of-plane (OOP) are often used interchangeably. Out of plane (OOP) refers to the fact the beam of the ultrasound is traveling in a plane that is perpendicular to the plane of the nerve or vessel.

Longitudinal scan

During a longitudinal scan, the probe is placed in the same plane as the target being imaged. The ultrasound beam travels along the long axis of the nerve or blood vessel. In a longitudinal scan, blood vessels and nerves appear as linear structures (Figure 3.8a and b).

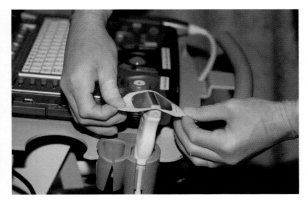

Figure 3.1 Sterile Tegaderm™ for single-shot blocks: placed tightly to eliminate any pockets of air between the probe and the Tegaderm™.

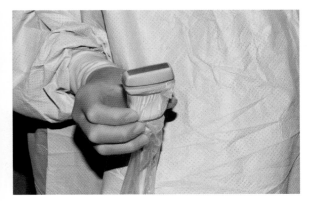

Figure 3.2 Sterile probe sheath used for perineural catheters: conduction gel placed inside the sheath to eliminate pockets of air between the probe and the sheath.

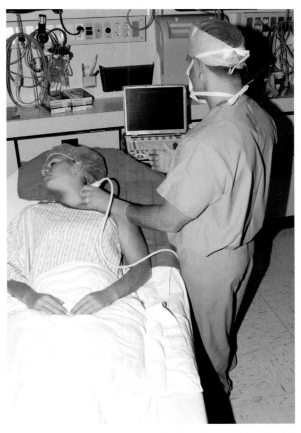

Figure 3.4 Proper positioning: the bed is at the correct height with the anesthesiologist's body braced against the bed, the elbow is against the body, the arm and hand are resting on the patient, the probe is gripped low to provide stability, and the ultrasound is placed near the patient's head.

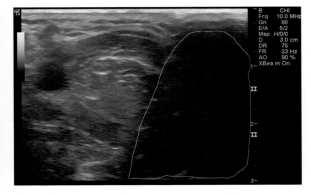

Figure 3.3 Anechoic artifact caused by pocket of air between the transducer and the patient.

The terms longitudinal, long axis and in-plane (IP) can be used interchangeably.

Transducer movement

Proper scanning to find target structures may require *large movements* and/or *small movements* of the probe. Large movements are movements of the probe that require the operator to move his/her shoulder or elbow. Small movements are movements of the wrist in order to fine tune the image. Remember that nerves exhibit anisotropy, meaning that their appearance can be either hyperechoic or hypoechoic depending on the angle of the ultrasound transducer to the nerve. Sometimes a small movement is all that is required to make an invisible hypoechoic nerve, which blends into the background, become an easily identifiable

25

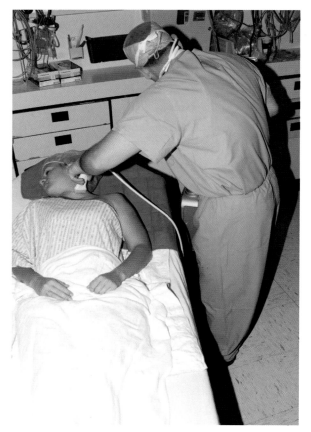

Figure 3.5 Improper positioning: the bed is too low forcing the anesthesiologist to hunch over, the anesthesiologist's body is not braced against the bed, the elbow is away from the body, the arm is not rested on the patient, the probe is gripped too high, and the ultrasound machine is placed such that the anesthesiologist is forced to rotate his body to view the image on the screen.

hyperechoic nerve. The sciatic nerve displays a great deal of anisotropy. Small angle changes can cause the sciatic nerve to come into view or disappear.

Systematic scanning

When performing an ultrasound-guided nerve block, a "systematic scan" of the target area should precede needle placement. The systematic scan for each block is a practiced set of scanning movements that allows an assessment of the immediate block area. Having a well practiced and rehearsed scanning process is important for a number of reasons. Systematic scanning:

1. Is important for the novice to reinforce anatomical relationships
2. Is important for more experienced practioners to survey the block area looking for occult dangers (e.g. blood vessels) or obstacles
3. Is important when facing patients with difficult or unusual anatomy.

Orienting structures

The orienting structure is a structure that can be easily identified and has a consistent anatomic relation to the target nerves being blocked. Normally the orienting structure is a blood vessel. Blood vessels are usually easy to identify and are anatomically close to the nerve plexus being blocked. Peripheral nerve blocks that do not have a blood vessel as the orienting structure will be more difficult to learn initially.

Normally the search for the orienting structure involves *large movements*. Once the orienting structure

(a)

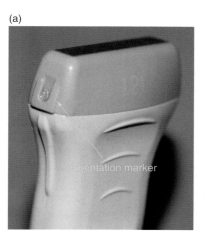

(b)

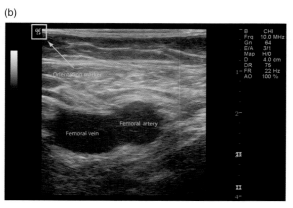

Figure 3.6 (a) and (b) Orientation marker on the ultrasound probe will correspond to the *GE* mark on the screen during a femoral nerve block.

(a)

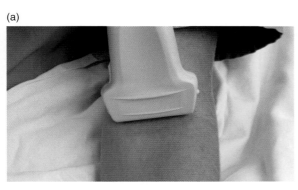

(b)

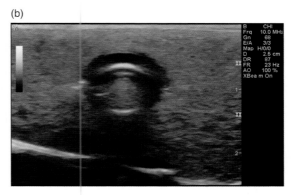

Figure 3.7 (a) and (b) Transverse scan: the probe is in a perpendicular plane to the nerve or vessel being imaged, yielding a rounded image of the vessel on the screen.

(a)

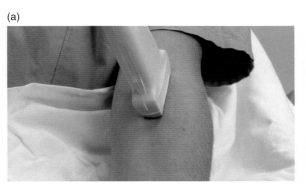

(b)

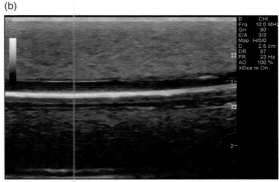

Figure 3.8 (a) and (b) Longitudinal scan: the probe is in the same plane as the nerve or vessel being imaged.

is found and the proximity of the target nerves is identified, then *small movements* of the wrist are used to fine tune the image. Once an image is obtained, it is crucial to hold the probe steady, hence the need for proper body mechanics as discussed earlier.

Needle insertion

In plane (IP)

The needle is inserted in the same plane as the ultrasound beam. The goal is for the path of the needle to be entirely within the beam of the ultrasound. The more parallel the needle is to the probe (shallower angle of insertion) the easier the needle will be to visualize (Figure 3.9a and b). When inserting the needle, the goal is to be as close to parallel to the probe as possible.

Since with many blocks it will be impossible for the needle to be parallel to the probe, the goal should be to have as shallow an angle of insertion as possible. In order to achieve a shallow angle between the needle and the probe, some blocks will require that the needle be inserted a greater distance from the probe as opposed to right next to the probe. Inserting the needle right next to the probe will cause a steep angle of insertion and can lead to poor needle visualization.

Partial plane

The width of the ultrasound beam is very thin, about the width of a credit card. When attempting an in-plane needle insertion, a small deviation will cause the needle to exit the ultrasound beam. Since only the part of the needle that passes in the ultrasound beam

27

(a) (b)

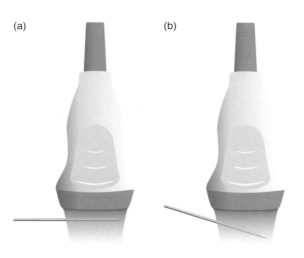

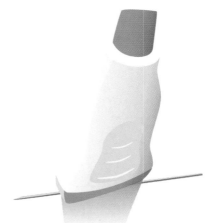

Figure 3.10 Partial plane: the tip of the needle is outside of the transducer beam. The true location of the needle tip is not known. The portion that appears as the tip of the needle is actually the middle of the needle.

Figure 3.9 (a) and (b) In-plane needle insertion: the more parallel the needle is inserted to the probe the easier it will be to visualize.

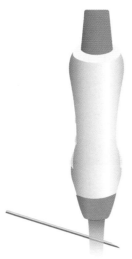

Figure 3.11 Out-of-plane needle insertion.

can be visualized, deviation from the ultrasound beam will cause loss of visualization of the needle tip. If the needle is partially within the beam and partially out, the part of the needle at the edge of the beam will appear as the tip of the needle (Figure 3.10). This can lead to a potentially dangerous situation as the physician will not know where the actual tip of the needle is. The partial-plane approach should be avoided.

Out of plane (OOP)

The needle is perpendicular to the beam of the ultrasound (Figure 3.11). The needle is seen as a small hyperechoic dot on the screen. In an OOP approach,

the needle needs to travel a shorter distance to the target than in an in-plane approach. For those making the transition from nerve stimulation to ultrasound, the location of needle insertion in the OOP approach is similar to the traditional nerve stimulator insertion points. Finding the needle tip in an OOP approach can be challenging for the beginner. The steeper the angle of insertion, the easier it is to see the needle in an OOP approach.

To avoid confusion, we will use the terms longitudinal and transverse when referring to scanning, and in plane (IP) and out of plane (OOP) when referring to needle insertion.

Local anesthetic injection

Once the proper location of the needle tip in relation to the target has been confirmed, local anesthetic injection can begin. Local anesthetic injected under ultrasound appears as an expanding hypoechoic region (Chapter 2). Injection of local anesthetic should be slow in order to avoid high injection pressures, which may lead to nerve damage. There are commercially available devices that monitor injection pressure. If there is high resistance to injection, the needle tip should be repositioned.

Monitoring local anesthetic spread is very important during performance of an ultrasound-guided nerve block in addition to other injection-safety practices. For example, it is important to gently aspirate prior to injection of local anesthetic and after each

(a)

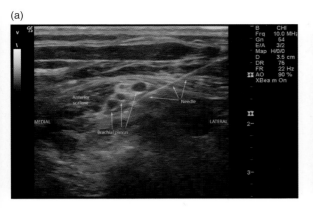

(b)

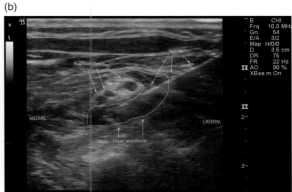

(c)

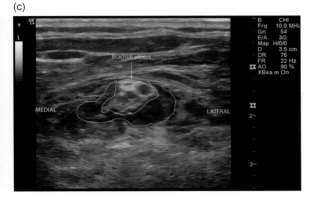

Figure 3.12 (a) Interscalene brachial plexus block with the needle placed next to the brachial plexus prior to start of injection. (b) Injection of local anesthetic has started and can be seen as an expanding hypoechoic region as outlined. (c) Injection of local anesthetic has been completed with the local anesthetic surrounding the brachial plexus.

needle movement, looking for blood return in the syringe. There are, however, case reports in the literature where seizure activity occurred following a negative aspiration with local anesthetic injection during an ultrasound-guided regional block. Therefore, a negative aspiration does not rule out the possibility of intravascular injection or subsequent local anesthetic toxicity. In theory, monitoring anesthetic spread around the nerve by ultrasound visualization should provide an additional safety feature, though this theory is unproven at the present time. Regardless, if the spread of local anesthetic cannot be visualized while the needle is in view, be alert to the possibility of an intravascular injection. Local anesthetic injected in a large vessel will give a hazy/smoky appearance.

In ultrasound-guided regional anesthesia, the pattern of local anesthetic spread is as important as the pattern of nerve stimulation is in nerve stimulator-guided regional anesthesia. Spread of local anesthetic around the nerves must be confirmed. Fascial planes and/or tissue surrounding nerves may keep the local anesthetic from reaching the nerve even if the needle is in close proximity to the nerve. If the local anesthetic is not reaching the target nerve, you must make small adjustments in order to surround the nerve with local anesthetic. Throughout this book we stress observing the pattern of spread rather than adhering to a fixed number of injections for a block, e.g., triple vs. single injection for an infraclavicular block. Complete coverage of a nerve or nerve plexus may require a single injection or it may require multiple injections. The need for good spread of local anestheisa must be balanced with the need to have as few needle passes as possible in order to minimize the chance for complications such as pneumothorax or nerve damage due to needle trauma. If multiple injections are required, try to minimize the number of passes and keep the needle movements as small as possible (Figure 3.12).

Although we advocate attempting to surround the nerve with local anesthetic, there are no studies to show this will lead to a more rapid onset, longer duration, or higher success rates. Our advocacy is based on anecdotal experience in our practice and assumptions based on anatomy and neurophysiology.

> **Key points**
>
> In ultrasound-guided regional anesthesia, the pattern of local anesthetic spread is as important as the pattern of nerve stimulation is in nerve stimulator-guided regional anesthesia.

Hydrolocation

Hydrolocation is the technique of using small injections of local anesthetic (0.5 to 1 ml) in order to visualize the tip of the needle. An area of expanding hypoechogenicity caused by injecting a small amount of local anesthetic can be helpful in confirming needle-tip position. While there are some patients for whom this technique may be a valuable aid, we do not advocate routine use of hydrolocation to locate needle tips. Beginners should concentrate on body mechanics, scanning, and needle insertion with a strict in-plane approach in order to visualize the needle tip in place of multiple blind injections (i.e., hydrolocation). Although hydrolocation is useful in locating the *tip* of catheters, and will be discussed in

the chapters on continuous catheters, hydrolocation should not be considered a substitute for proper technique.

Nerve stimulation

Nerve stimulation can be used as a confirmatory aid for those new to ultrasound-guided regional anesthesia. Nerve stimulation may be used in conjunction with ultrasound guidance as new blocks are attempted. Ultrasound-guided studies have shown the inability to elicit a motor response with a stimulating needle, even when the needle is in close proximity to the nerve. Therefore, as confidence is gained in the use of ultrasound for regional anesthesia, nerve stimulation can be abandoned in favor of a pure ultrasound-guided technique. Using nerve stimulation in conjunction with ultrasound guidance does not seem to improve onset times or success rates as compared to ultrasound alone.

Suggested reading

Beach M L, Sites B D, Gallagher J D. (2006). Use of a nerve stimulator does not improve the efficacy of ultrasound-guided supraclavicular nerve blocks. *J Clin Anesth*, 18(8):580–4.

Neal J M, Gerancher J C, Hebl J R, *et al.* (2009). Upper extremity regional anesthesia: essentials of our current understanding, 2008. *Reg Anesth*, 34(2):134–70.

Sinha S K, Abrams J H, Weller R S. (2007). Ultrasound-guided interscalene needle placement produces successful anesthesia regardless of motor stimulation above or below 0.5 mA. *Anesth Analg*, 105(3):848–52.

4

Upper extremity anatomy for regional anesthesia

The practice of regional anesthesia requires a sound understanding of anatomy. In the application of this knowledge, it is important to understand that although there are many consistencies in anatomy from one person to the next, there are also inconsistencies. Thorough knowledge and understanding of applied anatomy, as well as relative anatomy, will lay the groundwork for a successful practice of regional anesthesia. In this chapter, the basic anatomy for successful performance of regional anesthetic procedures for the upper extremity described later in this book will be introduced. In order to practice safe and successful upper extremity regional anesthesia, a fundamental understanding of the brachial plexus is necessary.

The brachial plexus

The brachial plexus (Table 4.1) innervates the skin and subcutaneous tissues (dermatomes), muscle (myotomes), and bone (osteotomes) of the entire upper extremity, with the exception of the axilla, and upper medial and some of the posterior arm (Figures 4.1 and 4.2). It primarily arises from the ventral rami of the C5 through T1 spinal nerves. Some variations may occur in which there may also be some contribution from either the C4 and/or T2 segments as well, but segments C5 through T1 comprise the consistent majority of the brachial plexus. As the brachial plexus travels from proximal to distal, it transitions from five *roots* to three *trunks* to six *divisions* to three *cords* and ends as five *branches*, which are the major terminal nerves of the brachial plexus (Figure 4.3).

The five roots, from C5 through T1, arise from their intervertebral foramina and travel caudal and lateral towards the first rib. Throughout this path they are enveloped by the posterior fascia of the anterior scalene muscle anteriorly and the anterior fascia of the middle scalene muscle posteriorly. These muscles have a proximal insertion from the C3 through C6 vertebrae and extend laterally to attach to the first rib.

As the brachial plexus roots course distally within this fascial envelope, they form the three trunks of the cervical plexus. The C5 and C6 roots combine to form the *superior* trunk, C7 continues as the *middle* trunk, and C8 and T1 join to form the *inferior* trunk. These trunks continue to travel distally toward the first rib, within the fascial plane formed by the anterior and middle scalene muscles. A key nerve to identify is the *suprascapular nerve*, which branches off the brachial plexus at the level of the trunks. It arises from the superior trunk and travels under the omohyoid muscle to the scapula where it passes through the superior scapular notch to innervate the supraspinatus and infraspinatus muscles as well as provide sensory distribution to the posterior aspect of the glenohumeral joint.

Once the trunks reach the lateral border of the first rib, all three trunks bifurcate into an anterior and a posterior division, forming the six divisions of the brachial plexus. In this region, the brachial plexus is anteriorly joined by the subclavian artery. From this point on, the brachial plexus will continue to travel distally to the terminal branches oriented around an artery.

As the brachial plexus continues to course distally, it enters the apex of the axilla, near the lateral border of the pectoralis minor. Here, the divisions combine to form the three cords of the brachial plexus. The anterior divisions of the superior and middle trunks (C5–7) combine to form the *lateral* cord. The anterior division of the inferior trunk (C8, T1) continues to form the *medial* cord. The posterior divisions of all three trunks (C5–T1) combine to form the *posterior* cord. The three cords of the brachial plexus are named for their orientation around what is now the axillary artery. Some key nerves that branch off at the level of the cords include the *medial brachial cutaneous* and *medial antebrachial cutaneous nerves*, which branch off the medial cord and supply the majority of the sensation to the medial arm, as well as the *musculocutaneous nerve*, which branches off the distal portion of the lateral cord.

31

Table 4.1 Summary of brachial plexus terminal nerve functions

Brachial plexus terminal branch	Cutaneous sensation	Joint sensation	Motor action
Axillary nerve (C5, C6)	Over deltoid muscle	Glenohumeral	Abduction of arm
		Acromioclavicular	Flexion of arm
			Extension of arm
			Lateral rotation of arm
Radial nerve (C5–T1)	Posterior arm and forearm	Elbow	Extension of arm
	Dorsum of hand	Radius–ulna	Extension and supination of forearm
	Dorsum of first three fingers and lateral half of fourth finger to DIP	Wrist	Extension of wrist, fingers, and thumb
			Abduction of thumb
Median nerve (C5–T1)	Thenar eminence	Elbow	Pronation and flexion of forearm
	Palmar surface of first three fingers and lateral half of fourth finger	Radius–ulna	Flexion of the wrist, fingers, and thumb
	Dorsum of first three fingers and lateral half of fourth finger distal to DIP	Wrist	Abduction of thumb
		Fingers	Opposition of the thumb
Musculocutaneous nerve (C5–C7)	Lateral aspect of forearm	Elbow	Flexion of arm
		Proximal radius–ulna	Flexion and supination of forearm
Ulnar nerve (C8–T1)	Hypothenar eminence	All in hand except thumb and ulna-carpal	Flexion of wrist and fingers, especially fourth and fifth
	Dorso-medial surface of hand		Adduction and flexion of thumb
	Dorsal and palmar surface of fifth finger and medial half of fourth finger		Opposition of fifth finger
			Spreading and closing of fingers

Once the cords extend into the axilla, just past the pectoralis minor muscle, the three cords form the five main terminal branches of the brachial plexus. The two main branches formed from the posterior cord are the *axillary nerve* (C5 and C6) and *radial nerve* (C5 through T1). Both the lateral and medial cords give off branches that join to form the *median nerve* (C5 through T1). Proximal to the branch to form the median nerve, the lateral cord gives off a branch as the *musculocutaneous nerve* (C5 through C7), while the medial cord continues as the *ulnar nerve* after it gives off its supplement to the median nerve. These are the five major terminal branches of the brachial plexus, but other nerves worth noting include the *thoracodorsal* and *subscapular nerves* from the posterior cord, the *lateral pectoral nerve* from the lateral cord, and the *medial pectoral nerve* from the medial cord.

- The *axillary nerve* is formed by fibers originating from the C5 and C6 levels. It travels with the posterior humeral circumflex artery and passes into the shoulder between the teres major and minor muscles and posterior to the humeral neck

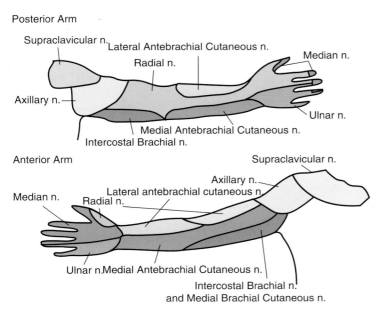

Figure 4.1 Sensory nerve distribution to upper extremity.

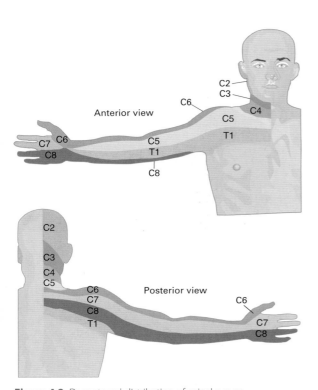

Figure 4.2 Dermatomal distribution of spinal nerves.

to innervate the teres minor and deltoid muscles, which can abduct, flex, extend, and laterally rotate the arm. It provides cutaneous sensation overlaying the deltoid, and provides sensation to the glenohumeral and acromioclavicular joints.

- The *radial nerve* is formed by fibers originating from the C5 through T1 levels. It travels with the deep radial artery along the spiral groove of the humerus, deep to the long head of the triceps, until it crosses the elbow anterior to the lateral epicondyle, between the brachialis and brachioradialis muscles. As it passes the elbow, it divides into a deep and superficial branch that continues distally down the forearm along the interosseous membrane and along the deep surface of the brachioradialis muscle, respectively. Several inches proximal to the wrist, it separates from the radial artery and passes into the wrist as multiple, small cutaneous branches in the region of the radial styloid and anatomic "snuff box" to enter the hand. The radial nerve innervates the three heads of the triceps brachii muscle, as well as many of the muscles involved in extension of the arm, extension or supination of the forearm, extension of the wrist, fingers, and thumb, and abduction of the thumb. It supplies cutaneous

33

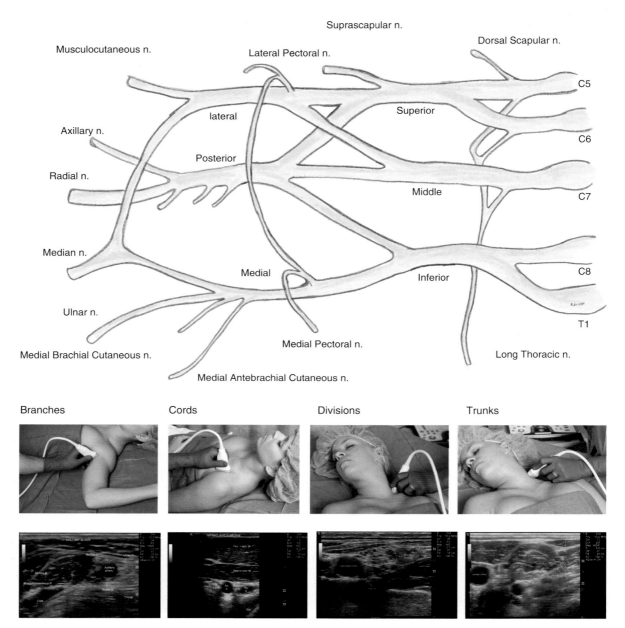

Figure 4.3 Brachial plexus with various peripheral nerves to upper extremity.

sensation to the skin covering the distal-lateral arm as the *inferior lateral brachial cutaneous nerve,* the posterior arm and forearm, the dorsum of the hand onto the first three fingers, and the lateral half of the fourth finger to the level of the distal interphalangeal joint, and provides sensation to the joints of the elbow, radius–ulna, and wrist.

- The *median nerve* is formed by fibers originating from the C5 through T1 levels. It travels with the brachial artery down the arm and crosses the elbow in the cubital fossa, medial to the artery, then continues down the forearm between the flexor digitorum profundus and superficialis muscles. At the wrist, it passes between the palmaris longus (laterally) and flexor digitorum (medially) tendons, deep to the flexor retinaculum, in what is commonly referred to as the carpal tunnel, to enter the hand. The median nerve innervates many of the muscles involved in pronation and flexion of the forearm, flexion of the wrist, fingers, and thumb, as well as abduction and opposition of the thumb. It supplies cutaneous sensation to the palm's thenar eminence and the palmar surface of the first three fingers and the lateral half of the fourth finger, wrapping over to also supply the posterior surface of the fingers distal to the distal interphalangeal joint, and provides sensation to the joints of the elbow, radius–ulna, wrist, and fingers.

- The *musculocutaneous nerve* is formed by fibers originating from the C5 through C7 levels. It pierces into the coracobrachialis muscle and travels down the arm between the biceps brachii and brachioradialis muscles, then becomes the *lateral antebrachial cutaneous nerve* at the level of the elbow. The musculocutaneous nerve innervates these three muscles, which are involed in flexion of the arm and flexion and supination of the forearm. It supplies cutaneous sensation to the lateral aspect of the forearm, and sensation to the joints of the elbow and proximal radius–ulna.

- The *ulnar nerve* is formed by fibers originating from the C8 and T1 levels. It travels down the arm with the brachial artery until it reaches the elbow where it separates from the artery and crosses the elbow posterior to the medial epicondyle, then continues down the forearm between the flexor carpi ulnaris and flexor digitorum profundus muscles. At the wrist, it passes over the ulnar styloid and lateral to the ulnar artery to enter the hand. It innervates several of the muscles involved in flexing the wrist and fingers, particularly the fourth and fifth fingers, opposition of the fifth finger, adduction and flexion of the thumb, and spreading and closing of the fingers by innervating all of the interosseous muscles in the hand. The ulnar nerve supplies cutaneous sensation to the hypothenar eminence, dorsal and medial surface of the hand, and the dorsal and palmar surface of the fifth and medial half of the fourth fingers, and sensation to all the joints of the hand except for the thumb and ulnocarpal joint.

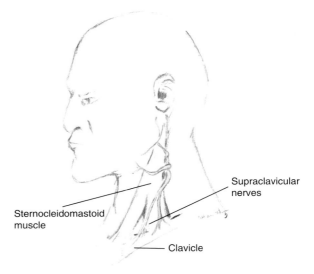

Figure 4.4 Superficial cervical plexus as it emerges from the lateral border of the sternal head of the sternocleidomastoid.

The cervical plexus

The cervical plexus innervates much of the skin, muscles, and bones of the anterior neck. It arises primarily from the ventral rami of the C2 through C4 spinal nerves. The plexus travels deep to the sternocleidomastoid muscle and gives off several branches superficially, forming the *superficial cervical plexus*, as well as deeply forming the *deep cervical plexus*.

The superficial cervical plexus supplies cutaneous sensation to much of the head, neck, and anterior shoulder. It has four main branches that penetrate through the cervical fascia, along the posterior border of the sternocleidomastoid muscle (Figure 4.4).

- The *lesser occipital nerve* is formed by fibers originating from the C2 and C3 levels. It travels superiorly then branches to supply cutaneous sensation to the superior and lateral area of the neck as well as much of the occipital region of the scalp.

- The *greater auricular nerve* is formed by fibers originating from the C2 and C3 levels. It travels anteriorly and superiorly then branches to supply cutaneous sensation to much of the ear and mastoid as well as inferior and posterior aspects of the face.

- The *transverse cervical nerve* is formed by fibers originating from the C2 and C3 levels. It travels

35

anteriorly and supplies cutaneous sensation to the anterior aspect of the neck.

- The *supraclavicular nerves* are formed by fibers originating from the C3 and C4 levels. They travel inferiorly and laterally and supply cutaneous sensation over the clavicle and anterior chest to the second rib, and provide sensation to the sternoclavicular and acromioclavicular joints.

The deep cervical plexus supplies input to the deeper structures of the neck. This input includes motor innervation to several muscles of the anterior neck that promote inspiration, such as the infrahyoid muscles and the scalene muscles. The deep cervical plexus also gives off a branch to the diaphragm as the *phrenic nerve*. It provides motor input to the diaphragm as well as sensation to both the inferior and superior surfaces of the diaphragm. It is formed from fibers from the C3 through C5 levels and travels down the neck along the anterior surface of the anterior scalene muscle into the mediastinum to the diaphragm.

Suggested reading

Netter F H. (2006). *Atlas of Human Anatomy*, 4th edn. Philadelphia: Saunders Elsevier.

Rohen J W, Yokochi C, Lutjen-Drecoll E. (2002). *Color Atlas of Anatomy: A Photographic Study of the Human Body*, 5th edn. Philadelphia: Lippincott Williams & Wilkins.

Sauerland E K. (1999). *Grant's Dissector*, 12th edn. Philadelphia: Lippincott Williams & Wilkins.

Chapter 5

Interscalene brachial plexus block

Introduction and anatomy

The interscalene approach involves blocking the roots and/or trunks of the brachial plexus. This approach is commonly used for postoperative pain control for procedures of the shoulder and arm, extending to the elbow.

Brachial plexus

The ventral rami of the C5 to T1 nerve roots come together to form the three trunks of the brachial plexus: superior, middle, and inferior. The superior trunk is formed by the C5 and C6 nerve roots, the middle trunk is composed of the C7 nerve root, and the inferior trunk is formed by the C8 and T1 nerve roots. In some individuals the superior trunk may have contribution from C4, and the inferior trunk may have contribution from T2 (Figure 5.2). The trunks of the brachial plexus travel between the anterior and middle scalene muscles (Figure 5.1). The anterior scalene muscle arises from the third or fourth to the sixth cervical vertebrae and takes a lateral course as it attaches to the first rib. The middle scalene muscle is the largest of the three scalene muscles as it arises from all of the cervical vertebrae, except the first or the first and second cervical vertebra, and also attaches to the first rib. Anatomic variations exist in many individuals. In some patients, the roots and/or trunks of the brachial plexus may pierce the anterior scalene muscle rather than travel within the interscalene groove (Figure 5.12). The phrenic nerve travels on the anterior surface of the anterior scalene muscle deep to the fascia of this muscle. The phrenic nerve courses behind the subclavian vein and into the thorax.

Suprascapular nerve

The **suprascapular nerve** is formed early from the superior trunk of the brachial plexus, and contains fibers from the C5 and C6 nerve roots. The nerve travels posteriorly through the suprascapular notch as it passes between the supraspinatus and infraspinatus muscles, providing motor innervation to these muscles as well as the posterior/superior shoulder capsule, glenohumeral joint, and the acromioclavicular joint (Figures 5.5 and 5.6). The supraspinatus muscle, which is inervated by the the suprascapular nerve, is the most commonly torn rotator cuff muscle.

Superficial cervical plexus

The cervical plexus is primarily formed by the ventral rami of C2 to C4. The plexus lies deep to the sternocleidomastoid muscle and gives off both deep and superficial branches. The superficial branches emerge from the lateral border of the sternocleidomastoid muscle to give four terminal branches: (1) lesser occipital nerve, (2) great auricular nerve, (3) transverse cervical nerve, and (4) the supraclavicular nerves. The supraclavicular branches provide sensation to the skin overlying the shoulder and clavicle (Figure 5.4). Local anesthetic from an interscalene nerve block will in most cases spread to the superficial cervical plexus. Some patients may require the superficial cervical plexus to be blocked separately.

> **Additional considerations**
>
> Proximal spread and/or the proximity of the phrenic nerve to the brachial plexus causes a nearly 100% concurrent block of the phrenic nerve with an interscalene brachial plexus block.
>
> Proximal spread of local anesthetic to the C2 to C4 nerve roots following an interscalene brachial plexus block can concurrently block the superficial cervical plexus.
>
> The nerve supply to the clavicle is primarily from two sources: (1) the *middle supraclavicular nerve*, which is a branch of the superficial cervical plexus, and (2) the

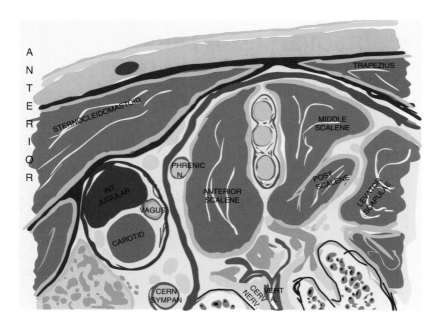

Figure 5.1 Cross-sectional representation of the neck for an interscalene brachial plexus block. Reproduced with permission of Jack Vander Beek. www.neuraxiom.com

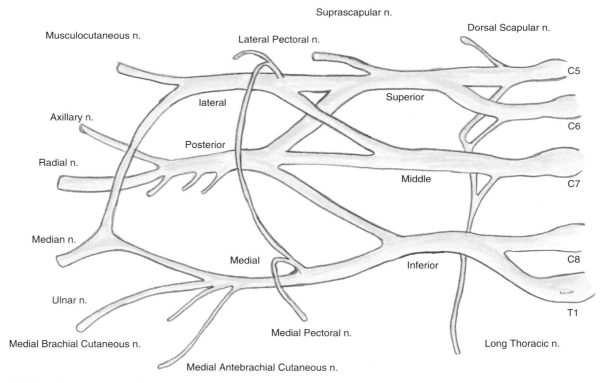

Figure 5.2 Brachial plexus with various peripheral nerves to upper extremity.

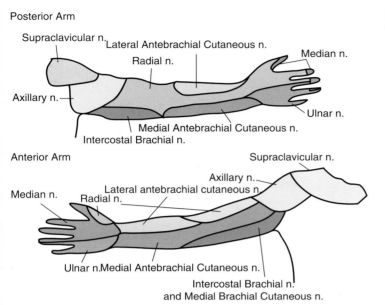

Figure 5.3 Sensory nerve distribution to upper extremity.

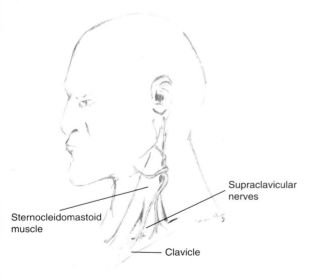

Figure 5.4 Superficial cervical plexus and its branches.

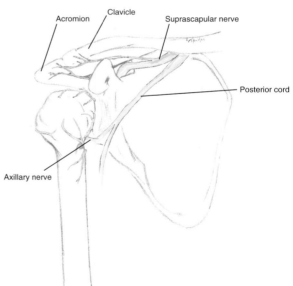

Figure 5.5 Anterior innervation of the shoulder.

nerve to the subclavius muscle, which is a small branch of the superior trunk of the brachial plexus.

Due to the early branching of the suprascapular nerve from the superior trunk of the brachial plexus, the nerve may be missed if the interscalene nerve blocked is performed too caudal on the neck.

Ultrasound anatomy
Interscalene region
Orienting structure: carotid artery

The carotid artery is seen as an anechoic pulsatile, non-compressible round structure. The internal

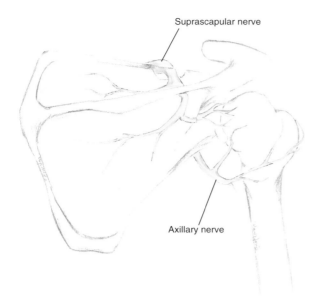

Figure 5.6 Posterior innervation of the shoulder.

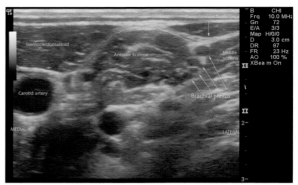

Figure 5.7 Ultrasound anatomy for a left-sided interscalene block with the carotid artery as orienting structure.

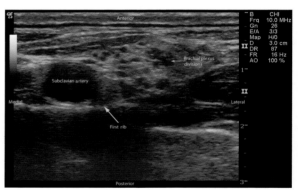

Figure 5.9 Ultrasound anatomy for a left-sided supraclavicular block with divisions of the brachial plexus lateral to the subclavian artery.

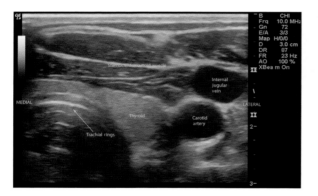

Figure 5.8 Scan carried out in the medial direction showing tracheal rings and the thyroid gland.

jugular vein is seen as an anechoic, non-pulsatile and compressible structure superficial to the carotid artery. The brachial plexus will appear as small round and/or oval hypoechoic structures traveling in the interscalene groove between the anterior and middle scalene muscles. The interscalene groove may correlate to a small dip in the deep cervical fascia (Figure 5.7). In some individuals the transverse process of cervical vertebrae and the vertebral artery may be seen. Scanning medially shows the thyroid gland and tracheal rings (Figure 5.8).

Supraclavicular region
Orienting structure: subclavian artery

The subclavian artery is seen as a large, non-compressible, round, and anechoic structure. The divisions of the brachial plexus are seen as small round to oval hypoechoic structures that may have a "honeycomb" appearance. Under two-dimensional ultrasound imaging, the brachial plexus will be seen superficial and lateral to the subclavian artery, or in the 1- to 3-o'clock or the 9- to 11-o'clock position, depending on whether left- or right-sided block is being performed. A bright hyperechoic line under the subclavian artery is the first rib (Figure 5.9). Familiarity with the ultrasound appearance of the structures listed below is recommended for successful interscalene brachial plexus block.

Table 5.1 Sample operative procedures for consideration of interscalene brachial plexus block

Procedure		Supplemental block
Arthroscopic shoulder procedures	R	Superficial cervical plexus
Open shoulder procedures	R	Superficial cervical plexus
Procedures involving the clavicle	R	Superficial cervical plexus
Proximal humerus	R	Intercostobrachial
Distal bicep repair	M	Intercostobrachial
Open/arthroscopic elbow	M	Intercostobrachial
Ulnar nerve transposition	M	Intercostobrachial
Hemodialysis access procedures (above the elbow)[1]	M	Intercostobrachial
Forearm[2]	NR	
Hand[2]	NR	

Notes: R = recommended; M = maybe; NR = not recommended.
[1] Some fistulas may cross the antecubital fossa.
[2] Field block of the intercostobrachial nerve will also provide coverage of the medial brachial cutaneous and medial antebrachial cutaneous nerves.

Sample operative procedures for consideration of interscalene brachial plexus block are shown in Table 5.1.

Structures that are required to be identified	Structures that may be seen
Carotid artery	Transverse process
Internal jugular vein	Thyroid
Sternocleidomastoid muscle	Trachea
Anterior scalene muscle	Vertebral artery
Middle scalene muscle	
Trunks/divisions of the brachial plexus	
Deep cervical fascia	
Subclavian artery	
First rib/pleura	

Contraindications

Contraindications to an interscalene brachial plexus nerve block are shown in Table 5.2.

Table 5.2 Contraindications to interscalene brachial plexus nerve block

Absolute contraindications	Relative contraindications
Patient refusal	Severe pulmonary disease
Infection over site of needle insertion	Ipsilateral neuromuscular disease/damage
Allergy to local anesthetics	Contralateral phrenic nerve/diaphragm damage
	Contralateral recurrent laryngeal nerve damage
	Anticoagulation or bleeding disorder
	Sepsis or untreated bacteremia
	Cervical hardware
	contralateral pneumothorax

Table 5.3 Side effects and complications associated with interscalene brachial plexus nerve block

Side effects	Complications[1]
Horner syndrome	Subarachnoid/epidural spread
Phrenic nerve block	Pneumothorax
Recurrent laryngeal nerve block	
Motor and sensory blockade of the arm	

Note: [1] Infection, nerve damage, vascular trauma, local anesthetic toxicity, and excessive bleeding are potential complications common to all nerve blocks.

Side effects and complications

Side effects and complications associated with an interscalene brachial plexus nerve block are shown in Table 5.3.

Horner syndrome

Horner syndrome is caused by the spread of local anesthetic to the cervical ganglion (Figure 5.1). Horner syndrome is manifested by ptosis, myosis, and anhydrosis on the ipsilateral side. Patients should be informed about the possibility of Horner

41

syndrome, as the signs and symptoms may be confused with a stroke. Incidence of Horner syndrome does not seem to be decreased by using lower volumes of local anesthetic.

Phrenic nerve block

The proximity of the brachial plexus to the phrenic nerve, and/or the proximal spread of local anesthetic to the nerve roots, causes the concurrent blockade of the phrenic nerve nearly 100% of the time. In healthy patients, phrenic nerve block is compensated by an increase in respiratory rate and increased effort by the intercostal muscles. Usually, healthy patients do not experience the subjective feeling of dyspnea; pneumothorax must be considered in a patient experiencing dyspnea following a peripheral nerve block above the clavicle.

Recurrent laryngeal nerve block

Unilateral recurrent laryngeal nerve block can lead to hoarseness, which can be bothersome to the patient but is benign.

Technique
Equipment

Ultrasound machine
High-frequency linear array probe
Sterile skin preparation
5-cm block needle
Ultrasound probe cover
Sterile ultrasound conduction gel
Local anesthetic for skin infiltration at block needle insertion site
Sterile gloves
Appropriate local anesthetic in 20-ml syringes

Scanning

Due to the shallow position of the brachial plexus in this region, ultrasound imaging of the brachial plexus is best accomplished by using a high-frequency linear array probe. A depth setting of 2 to 3 cm is usually adequate in the average person. The patient is positioned supine, the bed is raised so that it is level with the waist of the physician and the head of the bed is

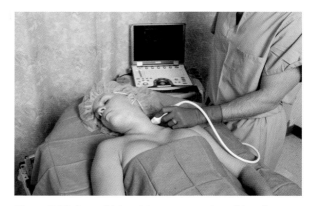

Figure 5.10 Scan with hand that corresponds to side to be blocked: place the ultrasound machine at the head of bed.

elevated between 30 and 45 degrees, with the ultrasound machine positioned at the head of the bed. The patient's head is turned away from the side to be blocked (Figure 5.10). The patient's neck is prepared from the ear to below the clavicle. The ultrasound probe is prepared with a sterile cover. A small amount of sterile conduction gel is applied to the tip of the sterile ultrasound probe. The probe is held in the hand that corresponds to the side to be blocked, thus for a right-sided procedure, the probe is held with the right hand, and for a left-sided procedure, the probe is held with the left hand. The probe should be oriented with the probe indicator to the patient's right. Scanning is performed in the transverse plane to the brachial plexus (Figure 5.11). The probe is placed on the neck to identify the carotid artery, which is the orienting structure for this block. The carotid artery will appear as a large, round, pulsatile, and non-compressible anechoic structure. Once the carotid artery is identified, slowly scan laterally to find the anterior scalene muscle. The trunks of the brachial plexus appear as three hypoechoic structures arranged in a cephalad to caudad direction between the anterior and middle scalene muscles in the interscalene groove (Figure 5.7). In some patients the trunks of the brachial plexus may travel within the anterior scalene muscle instead of within the interscalene groove (Figure 5.12). Color-flow Doppler and/or pulse-wave Doppler should be used to confirm the presence or absence of vascular structures since the roots/trunks of the brachial plexus in this region are hypoechoic and have a similar appearance to small vessels. The *transverse cervical, suprascapular,*

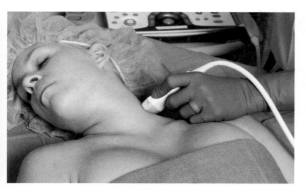

Figure 5.11 The hand is rested on the patient to provide a stable platform for scanning.

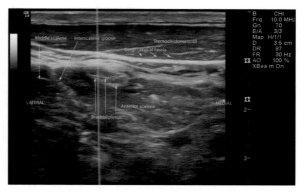

Figure 5.12 Brachial plexus passing through the anterior scalene muscle instead of the interscalene groove between the anterior and middle scalene muscles.

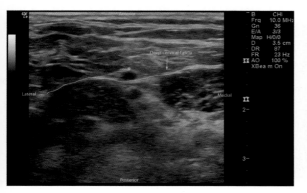

Figure 5.13 Notice the round hypoechoic structure above the deep cervical fascia.

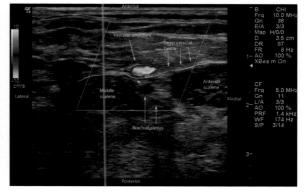

Figure 5.14 Color-flow Doppler identifying the structure as vascular.

or *ascending cervical arteries* may cross the brachial plexus in this region and should not be confused with the divisions of the brachial plexus and targeted for injection (Figures 5.13 to 5.16).

Additional considerations

A small "dip" in the deep cervical fascia may often correspond to the interscalene groove. The interscalene groove is between the anterior and middle scalene muscles and contains the brachial plexus.

Alternative scanning

In some patients, the identification of the brachial plexus and the scalene muscles may be very difficult.

Close proximity of nerves to an arterial structure, which is relatively easy to find with ultrasound, makes identification of nerves easier. Proximity to an easily identifiable structure narrows the area of focus and leads to faster and more accurate identification of the target nerves. The brachial plexus in the interscalene region lacks this close proximity to an arterial structure that makes its identification in some patients difficult. An alternative approach is to begin the scan in the supraclavicular fossa, similar to scanning for a supraclavicular block. In the supraclavicular fossa the brachial plexus has a close and consistent anatomic relationship with the subclavian artery, which can be readily identified with ultrasound (please refer to Chapter 6 for a complete discussion on supraclavicular blocks).

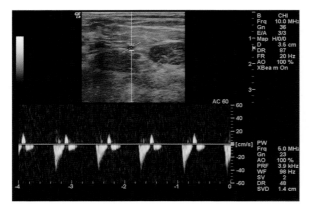

Figure 5.15 Pulse-wave Doppler is used to identify the structure as arterial.

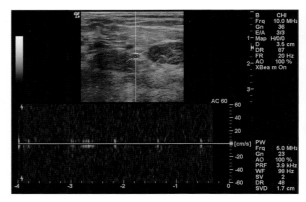

Figure 5.16 Round hypoechoic structure below the deep cervical fascia is identified as non-vascular.

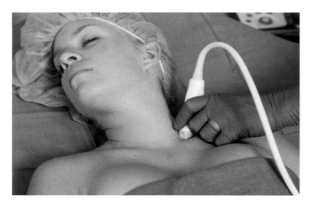

Figure 5.17 Start of scan: probe is placed in the coronal plane over the clavicle in the supraclavicular fossa.

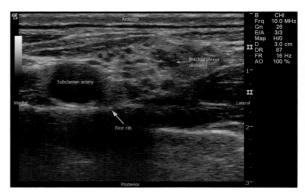

Figure 5.18 Large hypoechoic subclavian artery with a "honeycomb" consisting of small hypoechoic structures in the 2-o'clock position.

The probe is placed in the coronal plane above the clavicle, with the indicator to the right of the patient, in order to yield a transverse view of the subclavian artery (Figure 5.17). The subclavian artery appears as a large, non-compressible, anechoic structure. The divisions of the brachial plexus, under ultrasound, will appear cephalad and lateral to the subclavian artery as a cluster of hypoechoic structures, which may have a "honeycomb" appearance (Figure 5.18).

As the patient is scanned from caudad to cephalad, the divisions will slowly give way to the trunks of the brachial plexus. The scalene muscles and the interscalene groove are more prominent caudally, which will make identification of the scalene muscles easier. After the divisions of the brachial plexus have been identified, slowly scan cephalad. As the patient is scanned in the cephalad direction, the brachial plexus will move away from the arterial structure (subclavian artery). Take care to maintain visualization of the

divisions of the brachial plexus as the probe is moved cephalad (Figures 5.19–5.24).

Additional considerations

We recommend that all patients be initially scanned in the caudal to cephalad direction to gain experience with this technique and to serve as a confirmatory scan.

Needle insertion

After an adequate image is acquired, a small skin wheal is raised with local anesthetic near the lateral border of the probe. A blunt-tipped block needle is inserted in-plane (IP) with the probe, in a lateral to medial direction and directed towards the brachial plexus (Figure 5.25). A shallower insertion angle allows for greater reflection of ultrasound waves, and easier visualization of the needle as it passes under the

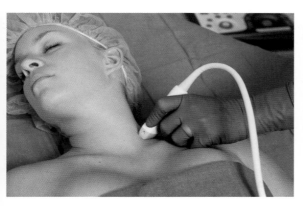

Figure 5.19 Scanning cephalad: probe is moved slightly more cephalad than in Figure 5.17.

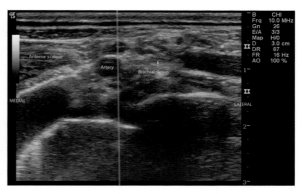

Figure 5.20 Anterior scalene muscle is starting to appear at the 9-o'clock position to the subclavian artery; the brachial plexus is still visible in the 2-o'clock position.

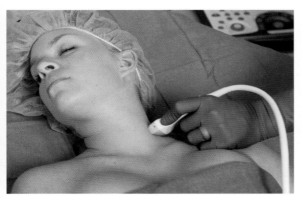

Figure 5.21 Probe is moved slightly more cephalad than in Figure 5.19.

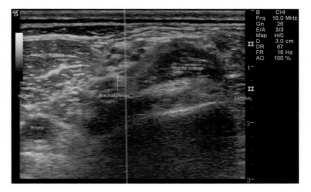

Figure 5.22 Anterior scalene is much more prominent now with the middle scalene starting to be seen. Notice separation of the brachial plexus from the orienting vascular structure. Effort must be made to maintain visualization of the brachial plexus in the middle of the screen.

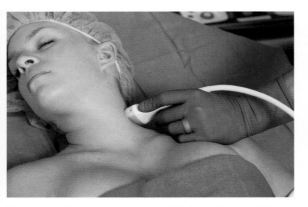

Figure 5.23 Probe is now more cephalad than in Figure 5.21 and in place for an interscalene brachial plexus block.

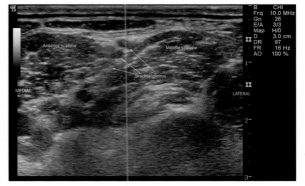

Figure 5.24 Divisions have given way to trunks: the anterior and middle scalene muscles can be clearly seen, as well as two trunks of the brachial plexus; small probe adjustments bring the third trunk into view.

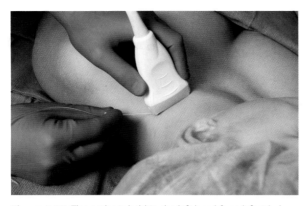

Figure 5.25 The probe is held in the left hand for a left-sided procedure; the needle is inserted in-plane with the ultrasound beam from a lateral to medial direction.

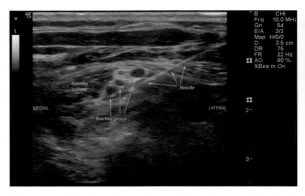

Figure 5.26 Block needle is advanced from the upper right-hand corner of the screen. The needle tip is located near the brachial plexus without making contact with the brachial plexus. This patient had a very small middle muscle.

probe. Look for the needle or tissue movement in the upper corner of the screen. Once the needle is under the transducer, it should become visible as a hyperechoic line. Do not blindly advance the needle. If the needle or tissue movement is not initially seen, make sure the needle is passing in the beam of the ultrasound probe. Small tilting or rotating movements of the probe may be needed to bring the needle into view. These movements should be small enough so that the initial image of the target structures changes minimally, if at all. If the original image changes significantly in order to locate the needle, this may indicate that the needle insertion was significantly off target, remove the needle and start over. It is safer, and more comfortable for the patient, to move the probe to find the needle than to move the needle in an attempt to see the needle under the probe. Seek the needle with the ultrasound beam instead of seeking the ultrasound beam with the needle. The needle is advanced through the middle scalene muscle, until the tip is located in the interscalene groove, near the brachial plexus without making contact with the brachial plexus (Figure 5.26). A "pop" may be felt as the needle is advanced through the middle scalene and into the interscalene groove. Care should be taken to avoid contacting the nerves of the brachial plexus in order to minimize the potential for nerve damage.

Additional considerations

A small insertion angle allows better visualization of the needle as the reflected ultrasound beams take a more direct path back to the transducer. Use the smallest needle insertion angle possible.

Local anesthetic injection

Once the needle is placed near the brachial plexus, injection of local anesthetic should be made slowly and with aspiration every 3 to 5 ml. If there is pain, paresthesia, and/or resistance during injection, stop and reposition the needle as this may indicate intraneural placement of the needle tip. The spread of local anesthetic should be monitored and will appear as an expanding hypoechoic region (Figure 5.27). The local anesthetic should surround the brachial plexus. If the local anesthetic is not spreading around the brachial plexus, the needle tip may be in the wrong fascial plane, which may require adjustment of the needle. Due to the fascial planes in this region, the needle tip may be in close proximity to the brachial plexus without getting adequate spread. Conversely the needle tip may be located far from the brachial plexus, but if the needle tip is in the correct fascial plane good spread of local anesthetic around the brachial plexus will be seen. The goal is to surround the brachial plexus with local anesthetic and not to just place the block needle close to the brachial plexus and inject (Figure 5.28).

Injection of local anesthetic may cause some neural structures to move. In order to completely surround the brachial plexus with local anesthetic, reposition the needle to better target the brachial plexus. However, the goal should be to minimize the number of needle passes in order to minimize the possibility of contacting the brachial plexus. Often a good spread can be achieved without having to reposition the needle. Aspiration should be carried out

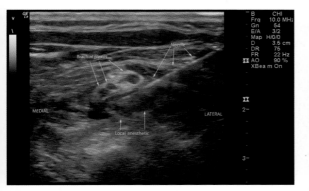

Figure 5.27 Local anesthetic beginning to spread around the brachial plexus.

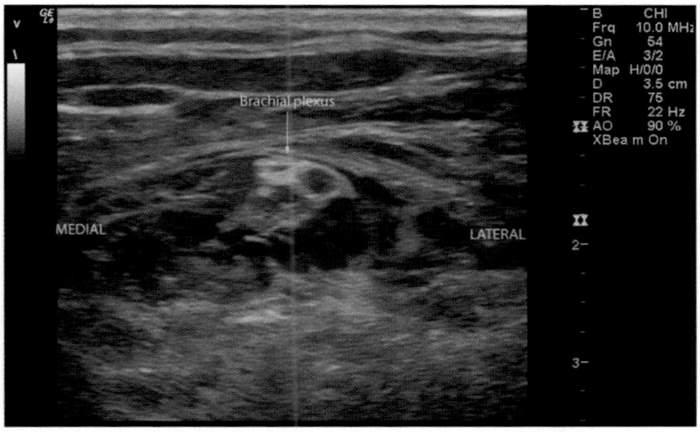

Figure 5.28 Local anesthetic spread around the brachial plexus at the completion of the block.

prior to injection after every change in needle position. Due to the differing acoustic impedance of local anesthetics, the needle, and tissue, once some local anesthetic is injected, the needle may become much easier to visualize.

One pitfall with this approach is the possibility of injection into the anterior or middle scalene muscles instead of injecting into the interscalene groove. Try to feel a "pop" as the needle passes through the fascia of the middle scalene muscle and into the interscalene groove. Make sure that the injection is deep to the deep cervical fascia as an injection of local anesthetic above the deep cervical fascia may not reach the brachial plexus. An injection into a large vessel may have a "smoky" appearance.

Additional considerations

A negative aspiration does not rule out an intravascular injection.

Remain alert to the possibility of intravascular injection if the spread of local anesthetic is not seen, as this may indicate that the local anesthetic is being deposited in a vessel and not perineurally.

Seizures may be caused by injection of small doses of local anesthetic into the carotid or vertebral arteries. Injection into these arteries will rapidly expose the brain to a high concentration of local anesthetic that may lead to a seizure.

Make sure that the injection is deep to the deep cervical fascia as an injection of local anesthetic above the deep cervical fascia may not reach the brachial plexus.

Authors' clinical practice

- *Dosing regimen*: we typically use 30 to 40 ml of 0.5% or 0.75% ropivacaine to provide postoperative analgesia for patients undergoing shoulder surgery. The volume and dose of anesthetic used will be influenced by the patient, patient's history, relevant comorbid conditions, and the spread of local anesthetic.

- It is important to cover the superior trunk as both the axillary (C5–C6) and suprascapular (C5–C6) nerves innervate the shoulder.

- We do not typically use a pure regional technique for shoulder surgery in the beach-chair position. Many patients cannot tolerate draping, the head holder, and the proximity of the surgical site to their head without sedation. We feel that the beach-chair position combined with extensive draping makes access to the airway more difficult should the need for airway manipulation occur. Also, a significant proportion of patients in the beach-chair position after interscalene block for shoulder arthroscopy can experience severe hypotensive and/or bradycardic events.

- Studies looking at the effect of using lower volumes of local anesthetic on diaphragmatic paralysis have shown inconsistent results. If avoidance of diaphragmatic paralysis is critical, an interscalene block is not recommended.

- In patients with severe pulmonary disease who may not tolerate hemidiaphragmatic paralysis, we may consider a supraclavicular block combined with a superficial cervical plexus block and a suprascapular nerve block. Although a

47

supraclavicular block also carries the risk of hemidiaphragmatic paralysis, the risk is lower and the effect on pulmonary function seems to be less. If hemidiaphragmatic paralysis is to be avoided completely, a superficial cervical plexus combined with a suprascapular nerve block can provide some analgesia for shoulder surgery without the risk of hemidiaphragmatic paralysis.

- Local anesthetic injected during an interscalene brachial plexus block may spread proximally to the C2–C4 nerve roots and block the superficial cervical plexus. The proximal spread from an interscalene block to the C2–C4 nerve roots may regress early and lead to early resolution of the superficial cervical plexus block. Therefore, we may perform a superficial cervical plexus block when the surgical procedure involves the clavicle or an open shoulder procedure.

- Posterior and/or anterior shoulder pain after arthroscopic or open shoulder surgery following a successful interscalene block may be due to shoulder capsule pain in the distribution of the suprascapular nerve or cutaneous pain from the superficial cervical plexus.

- Although we advocate attempting to surround the nerve with local anesthetic, there are no studies to support that this will lead to a more rapid onset, longer duration, or higher success rates. Our advocacy is based on anecdotal experience in our practice and assumptions based on anatomy and physiology.

- Classically, the interscalene brachial plexus nerve block has been used for above-the-elbow procedures. Studies using nerve stimulation alone have shown that in a substantial percentage of patients, the inferior trunk of the brachial plexus is not being blocked with an interscalene approach. If the inferior trunk is missed, the ulnar

nerve, the medial antebrachial cutaneous, and the medial cutaneous nerve will not be blocked; therefore, providing inadequate anesthesia of the medial portion of the arm, forearm, and hand. With ultrasound, it may be possible to visualize and block the inferior trunk of the brachial plexus. We do not use an interscalene block for surgery on the hand or forearm due to the unique risks and complications of interscalene blocks that are absent with more distal brachial plexus blocks.

Suggested reading

Borgeat A, Blumenthal S. (2007). Unintended destinations of local anesthetics. In: Neal J M, Rathmell J P (eds). *Complications in Regional Anesthesia and Pain Medicine*. Philadelphia: Saunders Elsevier, pp. 157–63.

Harry W G, Bennet J D C, Guha S C. (1997). Scalene muscles and the brachial plexus: anatomical variations and their clinical significance. *Clin Anat*, **10**(4):250–2.

Lanz E, Theiss D, Jankovic D. (1983). The extent of blockade following various techniques of brachial plexus block. *Anesth Analg*, **62**(1):55–8.

Neal J M, Gerancher J C, Hebl J R, *et al.* (2009). Upper extremity regional anesthesia: essentials of our current understanding, 2008. *Reg Anesth*, **34**(2):134–70.

Sinha S, Abrams J, Weller R S. (2008). Low vs. high volume ultrasound-guided interscalene block: pulmonary function and diaphragmatic motion. *Reg Anesth Pain Med*, **33**:A3.

Urmey W F, Gloeggler P J. (1993). Pulmonary function changes during interscalene brachial plexus block: effects of decreasing local anesthetic injection volume. *Reg Anesth*, **18**(4):244–9.

Urmey W F, McDonald M. (1992). Hemidiaphragmatic paresis during interscalene brachial plexus block: effects on pulmonary function and chest wall mechanics. *Anesth Analg*, **74**(3):352–7.

Chapter 6

Supraclavicular brachial plexus block

Introduction and anatomy

The supraclavicular brachial plexus block provides complete anesthesia or analgesia of the upper extremity and is carried out at the level of the distal trunks/ divisions of the brachial plexus. In the location that a supraclavicular block is carried out, the brachial plexus is in its tightest formation, thus allowing for rapid and complete anesthesia or analgesia of the upper limb. For this reason, a supraclavicular brachial plexus block has been called "spinal of the arm."

Brachial plexus

As the three trunks of the brachial plexus travel distally they divide into anterior and posterior divisions. The divisions sort the brachial plexus into the nerve fibers that are destined for the anterior and posterior aspect of the upper limb. The anterior divisions of the superior and middle trunk join to form the lateral cord. The posterior divisions of the superior and middle trunk join to form the major portion of the posterior cord (Figure 6.3). The inferior trunk continues as the medial cord after giving a small contribution to the posterior cord; this contribution may occur distal to the first rib.

The subclavian artery lies on top of the first rib and pleura with the divisions of the brachial plexus located cephalad and posterior to the artery (Figure 6.2). Of particular importance is the anatomic relation of the lung and the brachial plexus. The brachial plexus travels across the pleura of the lung prior to reaching the first rib and the subclavian artery; the apex of the pleura of the lungs extends into the base of the neck, rising 3 cm above the medial third of the clavicle and is level with the first thoracic vertebrae. The proximity of the brachial plexus to the pleura of the lung exposes patients to the risk of a pneumothorax.

The phrenic nerve arises from the third to the fifth cervical nerves. The phrenic nerve travels on the anterior surface of the anterior scalene muscle, deep to the

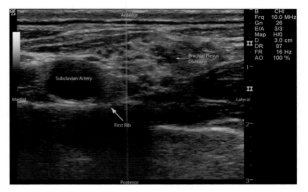

Figure 6.1 Left-sided supraclaviclar brachial plexus block: the brachial plexus at the 1-o'clock position.

Structures that are required to be identified	Structures that may be seen
Subclavian artery	Anterior scalene muscle[1]
First rib	Middle scalene muscle[1]
Divisions of the brachial plexus	Subclavian vein
	Bayonet artifact
	Mirror artifact
	Pleura

Note: [1]May be seen during a confirmatory caudal to cephalad scan.

fascia of this muscle, and enters the thorax by passing behind the subclavian vein. Occasionally the phrenic nerve may pass in front of the subclavian vein. The phrenic nerve can be blocked when performing a supraclavicular brachial plexus block, although the incidence is lower than with an interscalene block.

Ultrasound anatomy

The subclavian artery is seen as a large, non-compressible, round and anechoic structure (Figure 6.1 and

49

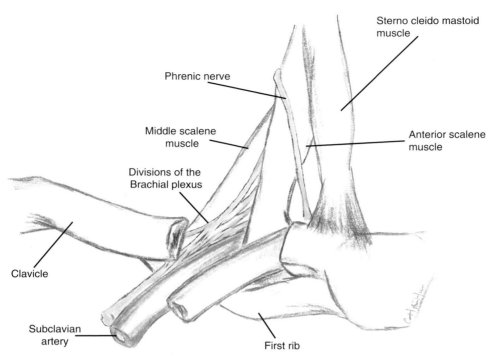

Sterno cleido mastoid muscle

Phrenic nerve

Middle scalene muscle

Anterior scalene muscle

Divisions of the Brachial plexus

Clavicle

Subclavian artery

First rib

Figure 6.2 Supraclavicular fossa anatomy. The brachial plexus and the subclavian artery travel across the pleura of the lung prior to reaching the first rib. The divisions of the brachial plexus are positioned cephalad and posterior to the subclavian artery.

Table 6.1). The divisions of the brachial plexus are seen as small round to oval hypoechoic structures that may have a "honeycomb" appearance. Under two-dimensional ultrasound imaging, the brachial plexus will be seen superficial and lateral to the subclavian artery, or in the 1- to 3-o'clock or the 9- to 11-o'clock position, depending on whether left- or right-sided block is being performed. A bright hyperechoic line under the subclavian artery is the first rib or pleura. Structures under the first rib will not be seen due to acoustic shadowing. Posterior angulation of the probe may show the subclavian artery and the brachial plexus lying on the pleura of the lung instead of the first rib. As the scan is carried cephalad, the anterior and middle scalene muscles come into view. The divisions of the brachial plexus can be very superficial as seen in Figure 6.1. The brachial plexus in this patient is less than 1 cm under the skin and less than 1 cm from the first rib.

Orienting structure: subclavian artery (Figure 6.1)

Table 6.1 provides sample operative procedures for consideration of supraclavicular brachial plexus block.

Contraindications

Table 6.2 lists contraindications to a supraclavicular brachial plexus nerve block.

Side effects and complications

Table 6.3 lists the side effects and complications associated with supraclavicular brachial plexus nerve block.

Horner syndrome

Horner syndrome is caused by the spread of local anesthetic to the cervical ganglion, and is manifested by ptosis, myosis, and anhydrosis on the ipsilateral side. Patients should be informed about the possibility of Horner syndrome, as the signs and symptoms may be confused with a stroke.

Phrenic nerve block

Although incidence of hemidiaphragmatic paralysis is lower following a supraclavicular block than an interscalene block, be alert to its potential. In healthy patients, hemidiaphragmatic paralysis is compensated

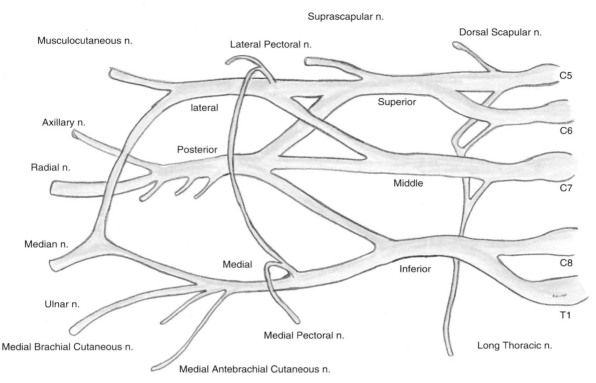

Figure 6.3 Brachial plexus with various peripheral nerves to upper extremity.

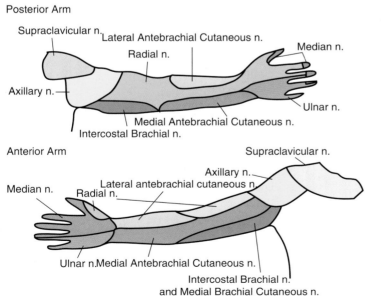

Figure 6.4 Sensory nerve distribution to upper extremity.

Table 6.1 Sample operative procedures for consideration of supraclavicular brachial plexus block

Procedure		Supplemental block
Procedures on the hand	R	–
Procedures on the forearm	R	–
Procedures on the elbow	R	Intercostobrachial
Distal biceps	R	Intercostobrachial
Hemodialysis access[1]	R	Intercostobrachial
Ulnar nerve transposition	R	Intercostobrachial
Open/arthroscopic shoulder procedures	M	Suprascapular, superficial cervical plexus
Proximal biceps repair	M	Intercostobrachial

Note: R = recommended; M = maybe; NR = not recommended.
[1]Some fistulas may cross the antecubital fossa.

Table 6.2 Contraindications to supraclavicular brachial plexus nerve block

Absolute contraindications	Relative contraindications
Patient refusal	Severe pulmonary disease
Infection over site of needle insertion	Ipsilateral neuromuscular disease/damage
Allergy to local anesthetics	Contralateral phrenic nerve/ diaphragm damage
	Contralateral pneumothorax
	Anticoagulation or bleeding disorder
	Sepsis or untreated bacteremia

Table 6.3 Side effects and complications associated with supraclavicular brachial plexus nerve block

Side effects	Complications[1]
Horner syndrome	Pneumothorax
Phrenic nerve block	Chylothorax
Motor and sensory blockade of the arm	

Note: [1]Infection, nerve damage, local anesthetic toxicity, and excessive bleeding are potential complications common to all nerve blocks.

by an increase in respiratory rate and increased effort by the intercostal muscles. Some studies have shown minimal change in spirometry values due to hemidiaphragmatic paralysis following supraclavicular nerve block. Usually, healthy patients do not experience the subjective feeling of dyspnea. In any patient experiencing dyspnea following a supraclavicular block, the possibility of a pneumothorax must be considered.

Pneumothorax

Due to the proximity of the divisions of the brachial plexus to the pleura, a supraclavicular nerve block carries a risk of pneumothorax. The rate of pneumothorax with ultrasound-guided supraclavicular blocks has not been well studied. Prior to the introduction of ultrasound to regional anesthesia, studies reported varying rates of pneumothorax with supraclavicular blocks. Although there is disagreement

about the validity of the reported rates of pneumothorax in some studies, there is agreement that due to the anatomic relationship of the brachial plexus and the lung in the supraclavicular fossa, the supraclavicular approach to the brachial plexus may carry a higher risk of pneumothorax than other approaches to the brachial plexus. A pnuemothorax can have a delayed presentation of up to 12 hours, especially in patients who did not have positive pressure ventilation.

Equipment
- High-frequency linear array probe
- Sterile skin preparation
- 5-cm needle
- Ultrasound probe cover
- Sterile conduction gel
- Lidocaine 1% for skin infiltration at block needle insertion site
- Sterile gloves
- Local anesthetic in 20-ml syringes
- Illustrated in Figure 6.5

Technique
Scanning

Due to the shallow location of the divisions of the brachial plexus, ultrasound imaging is best accomplished using a high-frequency linear array probe. A depth setting of 2 to 3 cm is usually adequate in

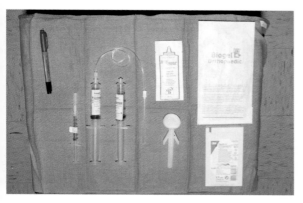

Figure 6.5 Equipment used for a superclavicular brachial plexus block.

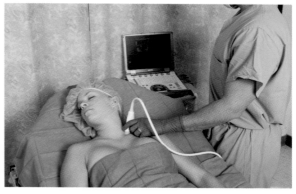

Figure 6.6 Positioning of the patient and ultrasound machine for a supraclavicular brachial plexus nerve block.

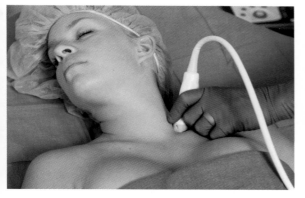

Figure 6.7 The probe is placed in the coronal plane, in a transverse orientation to the brachial plexus with indicator to the right of patient.

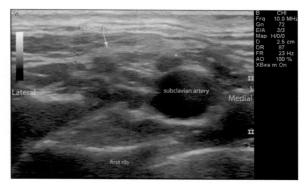

Figure 6.8 Shows a small round hypoechoic pulsatile structure next to the brachial plexus.

the average person. The patient is positioned supine with the head of the bed elevated between 30 and 45 degrees, and the patient's head is turned away from the side to be blocked (Figures 6.6 and 6.7). The patient's neck is prepared from the ear to below the clavicle. The ultrasound probe is prepared with a sterile cover and a small amount of sterile conduction gel is applied to the tip of the sterile ultrasound probe. The ultrasound machine is positioned at the head of the bed with the physician facing the patient. The probe is held in the hand that corresponds to the side to be blocked, thus for a right-sided procedure, the probe is held with the right hand, and for a left-sided procedure the probe is held with the left hand. The probe is placed in the coronal plane, above the clavicle, with the indicator to the right of the patient, in order to yield a transverse view of the subclavian artery (Figures 6.1 and 6.8). The subclavian artery

appears as a large, non-compressible, anechoic structure. The divisions of the brachial plexus are seen as small round to oval hypoechoic structures that may have a "honeycomb" appearance. Under two-dimensional ultrasound imaging, the brachial plexus will be seen superficial and lateral to the subclavian artery, or in the 1- to 3-o'clock or the 9- to 11-o'clock position depending on whether a left- or right-sided block is being performed. Once the subclavian artery and the brachial plexus are identified, slowly scan cephalad along the interscalene groove. The divisions of the brachial plexus should gradually give way to the three trunks of the brachial plexus, this will serve as confirmation and also allows practicing scanning for the interscalene block (please see Chapter 5 for a discussion of a caudal to cephalad scan for interscalene nerve blocks). Color-flow Doppler and/or pulse-wave Doppler should be used to confirm the presence or absence of

53

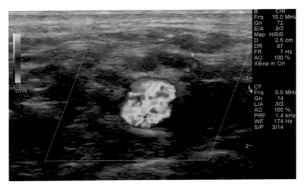

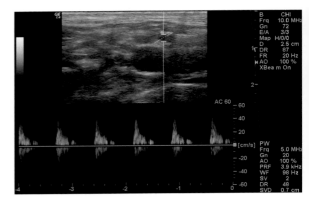

Figure 6.9 Color-flow Doppler used to confirm a structure is a blood vessel.

Figure 6.10 Pulse-wave Doppler used to show a structure is an artery.

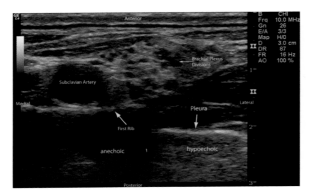

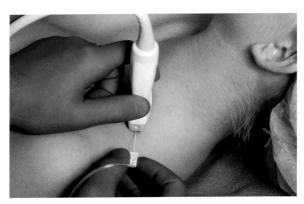

Figure 6.11 Two hyperechoic lines below the subclavian artery may represent the pleura and the first rib.

Figure 6.12 The needle is inserted in plane in a lateral to medial direction.

vascular structures since the divisions of the brachial plexus is this region are hypoechoic and have a similar appearance to small vessels (Figures 6.9 and 6.10). The *transverse cervical artery* and/or the *dorsal scapular artery* may cross the brachial plexus in the supraclavicular fossa and should not be confused with the divisions of the brachial plexus and targeted for injection.

Posterior angulation of the ultrasound probe may show the subclavian artery and the brachial plexus lying on the pleura of the lung as opposed to the first rib. Differentiating between the first rib and pleura can be difficult for the beginner. Due to strong attenuation by bone, areas behind the first rib are anechoic. However, the pleura may allow passage of some ultrasound waves, so the area distal to the pleura may be seen as a hypoechoic area (Figure 6.11). Whether the hyperechoic line below the subclavian artery is the first rib or the pleura, it represents an area of danger and should not be violated by the block needle.

Needle insertion

After an adequate image is acquired, a small skin wheal is raised with local anesthetic near the lateral border of the probe. A blunt-tipped block needle is inserted in plane (IP) with the probe in a lateral to medial direction and directed towards the brachial plexus (Figure 6.12). A shallow insertion angle allows for greater reflection of ultrasound waves, and easier visualization of the needle as it passes under the probe. Look for the needle or tissue movement in the upper corner of the screen. Once the needle is under the transducer, it should become visible as a hyperechoic line. Do not blindly advance the needle. If the needle or tissue movement is not initially seen, make sure the needle is passing in the narrow beam of the ultrasound probe. You may need to make small tilting or rotating movements with the probe to bring the needle into view. These movements should be small enough so that the initial image of the target structures should change minimally, if at all. If the original image changes significantly in order to locate the needle, this may indicate that the needle insertion was significantly off target, remove the needle and start over. It is safer, and more comfortable for the patient, to move the probe to find the needle than to move the needle in an attempt to see the needle under the probe. Seek the needle with the ultrasound beam instead of seeking the ultrasound beam with the needle. The ability to visualize the first rib in relation to the brachial plexus may give a false sense of security when performing this block. Due to the proximity of the brachial plexus to the first rib and the pleura, the margin of error is very small in some patients (Figure 6.1); therefore, it is important to maintain visualization of the tip of the needle at all times. Care must be taken to maintain a true *in-plane* view as opposed to a *partial-plane* view. A *partial-plane* view will give a false sense of security as to the true position of the needle tip and may cause the needle to be inserted too deep. Advance the needle until it is positioned beneath the brachial plexus and above the first rib (Figure 6.14). Care should be taken to avoid contacting the nerves of the brachial plexus in order to minimize the potential for nerve damage.

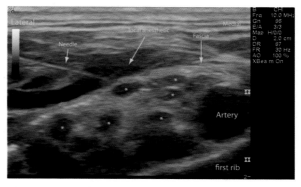

Figure 6.13 Local anesthetic injection is above a fascial plane and may not reach the brachial plexus even though the tip of the needle is in close proximity to the brachial plexus.

> ### Additional considerations
>
> A shallow insertion angle allows better visualization of the needle as the reflected ultrasound beams take a more direct path back to the transducer. Use the smallest needle insertion angle possible.
>
> Maintain the needle in the plane of the ultrasound beam. Avoid a *partial-plane* insertion of the needle.
>
> Seek the needle with the ultrasound beam instead of seeking the ultrasound beam with the needle.

Local anesthetic injection

Once the needle is placed between the brachial plexus and the first rib, the injection should be made slowly and with aspiration every 3 to 5 ml. If there is pain, paresthesia, and/or resistance during injection, stop and reposition the needle as this may indicate intraneural placement of the needle tip. The injection of local anesthetic must be in the correct fascial plane in order to surround the brachial plexus. The spread of local anesthetic should be monitored and will appear as an expanding hypoechoic region. If the local anesthetic is not spreading around the brachial plexus, the needle tip may be in the wrong fascial plane, which may require movement of the needle. Due to the fascial planes in the supraclavicular fossa, the needle tip may be very close to the brachial plexus without getting adequate spread of local anesthetic (Figure 6.13). Conversely the needle tip may be located far from the brachial plexus, but if it is in the correct fascial plane, a good spread of local anesthetic around the brachial plexus will be seen. The goal is to surround the brachial plexus with local anesthetic, not just to place the block needle close to the brachial plexus and inject.

Injection of local anesthetic may cause some neural structures to move (Figure 6.15). In order to completely surround the brachial plexus with local anesthetic, reposition the needle to better target the brachial plexus. However, the goal should be to minimize the number of needle passes to minimize the possibility of contacting the brachial plexus, the pleura, or blood vessels. Often a good spread can be achieved without having to reposition the needle. Aspiration should be carried out prior to injection after every change in needle position. An injection into a large vessel may have a "smokey" appearance.

> ### Additional considerations
>
> Due to the differing acoustic impedance of local anesthetics, tissue, and the needle, once some local anesthetic is injected, the needle may become easier to visualize.
>
> A negative aspiration does not rule out an intravascular injection.
>
> Remain alert to the possibility of intravascular injection if the spread of local anesthetic is not seen, as this may indicate that the local anesthetic is being deposited in a vessel and not perineurally.

55

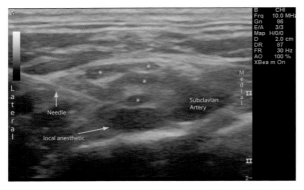

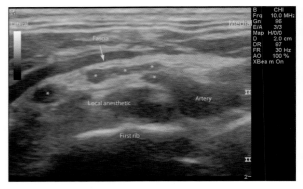

Figure 6.14 Needle repositioned deep to the fascia and local anesthetic injection is carried out below the brachial plexus and above the first rib.

Figure 6.15 Spread of local anesthetic at the completion of the block has compressed the brachial plexus and pushed it against the fascia.

Authors' clinical practice

- *Dosing regimen:* we typically use 30 to 40 ml ropivacaine 0.75% to provide surgical analgesia for patients undergoing orthopedic surgery. The volume and dose of anesthetic used will be influenced by the patient, patient's history, relevant comorbid conditions and the spread of local anesthetic.
- Use of shorter acting agents, such as mepivacaine or lidocaine, in place of ropivacaine may be more appropriate in situations when surgical anesthesia may be desired without postoperative analgesia (arteriovenous fistula), when early neurologic assessment postoperatively is required, or when patients desire early return of sensation or function to the blocked extremity.
- We do not routinely use a supraclavicular block for hand or forearm surgery due to the possibility of phrenic nerve block and risk of pneumothorax. When possible we use an infraclavicular block for hand and forearm surgery. The delay in presentation of a pneumothorax must be considered when selecting a supraclavicular block for outpatient surgery.
- If a supraclavicular nerve block is selected in patients undergoing shoulder surgery, we will supplement with a superficial cervical plexus and a suprascapular nerve block. Posterior and/or anterior shoulder pain may be due to shoulder capsule pain from the suprascapular nerve or cutaneous pain from supraclavicular nerve of the superficial cervical plexus.

- Although we advocate attempting to surround the nerve with local anesthetic, there are no studies to support that this will lead to a more rapid onset, longer duration, or higher success rates. Our advocacy is based on anecdotal experience in our practice and assumptions based on anatomy and physiology.
- We do not use a medial to lateral needle insertion. Although in a medial to lateral insertion the needle is being directed away from the lung, it is being directed towards the subclavian artery. The position of the subclavian artery may make reaching the brachial plexus difficult. Also, the position of the patient's head and neck relative to the probe and needle may make a medial to lateral needle insertion logistically more difficult.
- When training new residents we emphasize a very shallow needle insertion angle. For trainees who initially have difficulty in finding their needle, it is better to be too shallow than too deep. With a shallow insertion angle, if the needle is not immediately apparent and still advanced, the likelihood of violating the pleura or subclavian artery will be lower.
- An intercostobrachial nerve block may be used to alleviate some of the cutaneous discomfort associated with a tourniquet. True tourniquet pain is complex and partially due to muscle ischemia and will not be alleviated by this cutaneous block. However, block of the cutaneous nerves may aid in the intraoperative management of the patient if a purely regional technique is used.

Suggested reading

Borgeat A, Blumenthal S. (2007). Unintended destinations of local anesthetics. In: Neal J M, Rathmell J P (eds). *Complications in Regional Anesthesia and Pain Medicine*. Philadelphia: Saunders Elsevier, pp. 157–63.

Neal J M, Gerancher J C, Hebl J R, *et al.* (2009). Upper extremity regional anesthesia: essentials of our current understanding, 2008. *Reg Anesth*, **34**(2):134–70.

Neal J M, Moore J M, Kopacz D J, *et al.* (1998). Quantitative analysis of respiratory, motor, and sensory function after supraclavicular block. *Anesth Analg*, **86**(6):1239–44.

Perlas A, Lobo G, Lo N, *et al.* (2009). Ultrasound-guided supraclavicular block: outcome of 510 consecutive cases. *Reg Anesth*, **34**(2):171–6.

Urmey W F. (2007). Pulmonary complications. In: Neal J M, Rathmell J P (eds). *Complications in Regional Anesthesia and Pain Medicine*. Philadelphia: Saunders Elsevier, pp. 147–56.

Infraclavicular brachial plexus block

Introduction and specific anatomy
Brachial plexus

The ultrasound-guided infraclavicular brachial plexus block is carried out at the level of the cords. It is an excellent block for providing either surgical anesthesia or postoperative analgesia for all distal upper extremity procedures (Figures 7.2 and 7.3). This block is typically performed at the anterior shoulder and chest wall, in the area of the deltopectoral groove. At this site, the three cords of the brachial plexus travel distally, in close proximity to the axillary artery, from just below the clavicle to the axilla (Figure 7.4). The cords are named for their relative positions around the axillary artery as the lateral, posterior, and medial cords. These three cords will then divide and combine to form the five main terminal nerve branches of the brachial plexus. The posterior cord divides near the axilla to form the two main nerves of the axillary nerve and radial nerve. The lateral cord gives off a branch as the musculocutaneous nerve, branching off high in the axilla (sometimes arising within the level of the cords), then the remaining portion of the cord continues to become part of the median nerve. The medial cord gives off a branch as the ulnar nerve, and then continues to join the terminal branch of the lateral cord to form the median nerve. More proximally, the medial cord gives off two small branches high in the axilla (around the level of the branching of the musculocutaneous nerve from the lateral cord) as the medial brachial cutaneous nerve and the medial antebrachial cutaneous nerve. These supply the majority of the sensory innervation to the medial arm.

Additional considerations

Due to their branching high in the axilla, it is possible that some or all of the musculocutaneous, medial brachial cutaneous, and medial antebrachial cutaneous nerves may be spared when performing an infraclavicular block.

Intercostobrachial nerve

The intercostobrachial nerve arises primarily from the T2 intercostal nerve, with occasional supply from T1 or T3. Thus, it is not a component of the brachial plexus and is not anesthetized by a brachial plexus block. Along with the medial brachial cutaneous nerve, the intercostobrachial nerve provides sensory innervation to the axilla, as well as the upper medial and posterior arm (Figure 7.2).

Additional considerations

Procedures where the incision extends into the region of the upper medial arm may require a block of the intercostobrachial nerve.

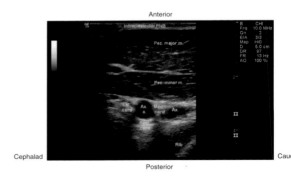

Figure 7.1 Normal infraclavicular ultrasound anatomy at the deltopectoral groove.

Structures that are required to be identified	Structures that may be seen
Axillary artery Axillary vein Cords of brachial plexus	Pectoralis major muscle Pectoralis minor muscle Rib/lung Anomalous vasculature

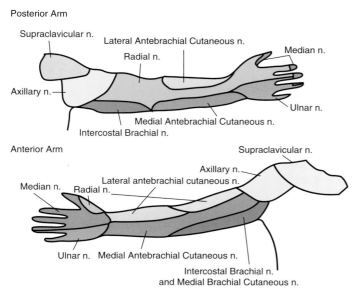

Figure 7.2 Cutaneous innervation of the upper extremity.

Posterior Arm

Supraclavicular n.

Lateral Antebrachial Cutaneous n.

Radial n.

Median n.

Axillary n.

Ulnar n.

Medial Antebrachial Cutaneous n.

Intercostal Brachial n.

Anterior Arm

Supraclavicular n.

Axillary n.

Lateral antebrachial cutaneous n.

Median n.

Radial n.

Ulnar n.

Medial Antebrachial Cutaneous n.

Intercostal Brachial n.
and Medial Brachial Cutaneous n.

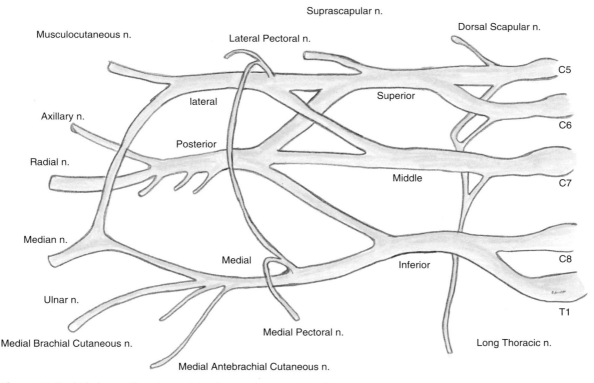

Suprascapular n.

Musculocutaneous n.

Lateral Pectoral n.

Dorsal Scapular n.

C5

lateral

Superior

Axillary n.

C6

Posterior

Radial n.

Middle

C7

Median n.

Medial

Inferior

C8

Ulnar n.

T1

Medial Brachial Cutaneous n.

Medial Pectoral n.

Long Thoracic n.

Medial Antebrachial Cutaneous n.

Figure 7.3 Brachial plexus with various peripheral nerves to upper extremity.

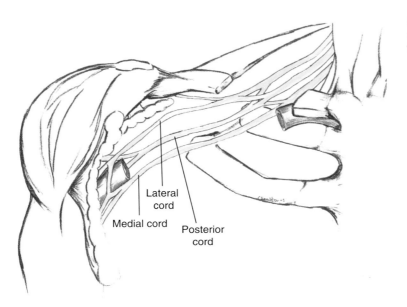

Figure 7.4 Dissection of the brachial plexus, showing position of cords at the deltopectoral groove.

Lateral cord

Medial cord   Posterior cord

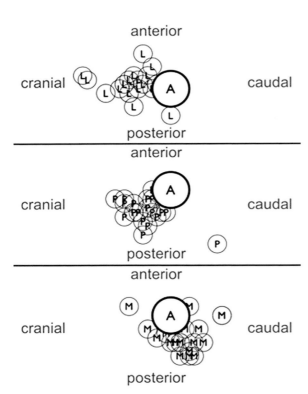

Figure 7.5 Anatomic variations of the infraclavicular anatomy in the coracoid region. Reproduced with permission from Sauter A R, Smith H-J, Stubhaug A, Dodgson M S and Klaastad Ø (2006). Use of magnetic resonance imaging to define the anatomical location closest to all three cords of the infraclavicular brachial plexus. *Anesth Analg.* 103(6):1574–6.

Ultrasound anatomy

Orienting structure: axillary artery

The orienting structure to perform this block is the *axillary artery* (Figure 7.1). At the site where the scanning and procedure are performed, the ultrasound image will show the lateral cord positioned cephalad to the axillary artery, the posterior cord positioned posterior, and the medial cord positioned caudad to the artery. In patients with normal relative anatomy, the medial cord is typically positioned in the small space between the axillary artery and vein. Although there may be variability in the exact location of these structures around the axillary artery (Figure 7.5), the three cords are typically located at approximately 3-o'clock, 6-o'clock, and 9-o'clock around the artery. Proper scanning and knowledge of the relative anatomy near the targets for this block are important in this region. The nearby vascular structures of the axillary artery and vein are consistently present, as well as the often closely oriented rib and pleura.

> **Additional considerations**
>
> Typically, the more medially one scans, the closer the proximity of the pleura to the brachial plexus.
>
> Anomalous vasculature is not uncommon in the infraclavicular region. Pay close attention to identifying any unknown hypoechoic structures, especially when they are in close proximity to the target structures or in the anticipated path of the needle.

Table 7.1 Sample operative procedures for consideration of infraclavicular brachial plexus block

Procedure		Supplemental block
Procedures of the hand and fingers[1]	R	–
Procedures of the wrist and distal radius[1]	R	–
Procedures of the forearm[1]	R	–
Hemodialysis access procedure below the elbow[1]	R	–
Distal biceps repair	M	Intercostobrachial nerve
Open/arthroscopic elbow	M	Intercostobrachial nerve
Ulnar nerve transposition	M	Intercostobrachial nerve
Procedures of the distal humerus	M	Intercostobrachial nerve
Hemodialysis access procedures (above the elbow)[2]	NR	–
Procedures of the proximal humerus/shoulder	NR	–

Notes: R = recommended; M = maybe; NR = not recommended.
[1]This block is useful for essentially any procedure or acute pain below the elbow.
[2]Some fistulas may cross the antecubital fossa.

Table 7.2 Contraindications to infraclavicular brachial plexus block

Absolute contraindications	Relative contraindications
Patient refusal	Ipsilateral neuromuscular disease/damage
Infection over site of needle insertion	Anticoagulation or bleeding disorder
Allergy to local anesthetic	Sepsis or untreated bacteremia

Table 7.1 shows sample operative procedures for consideration of infraclavicular brachial plexus block.

Table 7.3 Side effects and complications associated with infraclavicular brachial plexus block

Side effects	Complications[1]
Motor blockade of arm for duration of local anesthetic effect	Pneumothorax[2]

Notes: [1]Infection, nerve damage, local anesthetic toxicity, vascular injury, and excessive bleeding or hematoma are potential complications common to all nerve blocks.
[2]The close proximity of the rib and pleura to the target structures, especially when scanning or advancing the needle more medially, can lead to an inadvertent pleural puncture with a possible pneumothorax.

Contraindications

Table 7.2 lists contraindications to an infraclavicular brachial plexus block.

Side effects and complications

Table 7.3 lists some side effects and complications associated with infraclavicular brachial plexus block.

Equipment

- Ultrasound machine
- High-frequency linear array ultrasound probe[1]
- Sterile skin preparation
- 8- to 10-cm blunt-tipped needle (5-cm needle may be adequate for very small patients)
- Ultrasound probe cover
- Sterile ultrasound gel
- Local anesthetic for skin infiltration at block needle insertion site
- Sterile gloves
- Appropriate local anesthetic and volume in 20-ml syringes
- Illustrated in Figure 7.6

[1] Depending on the size (muscle mass and subcutaneous tissue) of the patient, the target structures may be fairly superficial (~2 cm) to fairly deep (~6 to 8 cm). When encountering a patient with very deep structures, a low-frequency probe may be beneficial. However, a high-frequency probe will be appropriate for most patients.

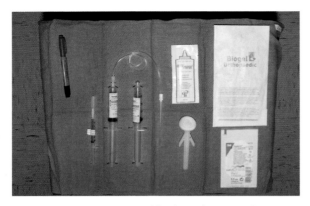

Figure 7.6 Equipment required for the performance of ultrasound-guided infraclavicular brachial plexus block.

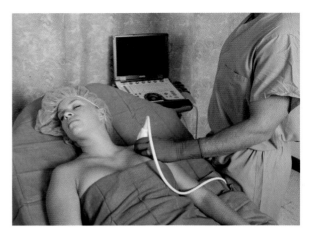

Figure 7.7 Proper positioning for scanning at the infraclavicular region.

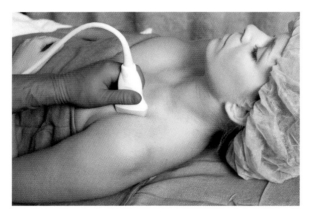

Figure 7.8 Proper ultrasound probe positioning for scanning at the infraclavicular region.

Technique

Technique summary

1. Monitors placed and patient appropriately sedated
2. Sterile preparation applied to procedural site
3. Clear Tegaderm™ applied to ultrasound probe
4. Perform systematic ultrasound scan to find optimal location for placement of nerve block
5. Skin wheal is raised
6. Insert block needle and guide towards target structures
7. Inject local anesthetic
8. Reposition needle as necessary

Scanning

The patient should be positioned supine, with the patient lying flat, or the head of the bed slightly elevated. The patient's arm should be held at his/her side, and his/her head should ideally be turned away from the extremity to be blocked. The ultrasound machine should be located near the head of the patient's bed, so that the screen is in an optimal viewing position for the physician, and the ultrasound controls are comfortably within the physician's reach. The physician performing the procedure should be positioned on the patient's operative side with his/her body facing the patient and his/her head turned to see the ultrasound screen. The height of the bed is adjusted so that the patient's deltopectoral groove is located in front of the physician's mid abdomen. The hand closest to the patient should control the ultrasound probe (Figure 7.7). A wide, sterile preparation is applied to the region of the deltopectoral groove, and sufficient ultrasound gel is applied to the site or probe to ensure adequate imaging.

The ultrasound probe is positioned along the *sagittal* plane over the deltopectoral groove (Figure 7.7, Figure 7.8), so that one end of the probe is oriented cephalad (corresponding to the orientation marker on the ultrasound screen) and the other end is oriented caudad. This will yield an ultrasound image in the transverse plane to the target structures. The depth of the scan and the position of the ultrasound probe should be adjusted (large movements) as needed in order to locate the pulsing axillary artery. This is the *orienting structure*, thus it should be the first structure identified when scanning for this procedure. Once this has been identified, the probe should be minimally tilted and rotated (small movements) in

(a)

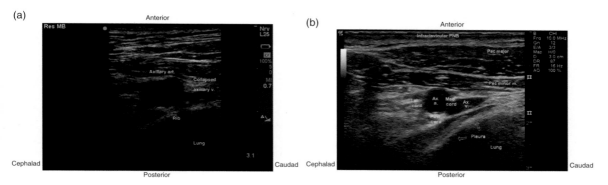

(b)

Figure 7.9 (a) and (b) Infraclavicular region showing potential proximity of cords to first rib and pleura.

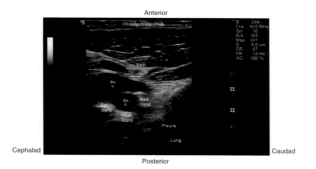

Figure 7.10 Infraclavicular region showing anomalous vasculature in potential path of the needle.

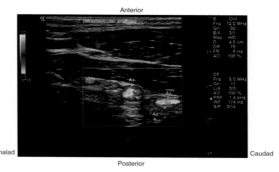

Figure 7.11 Infraclavicular region showing use of color-flow Doppler to identify anomalous vascular structures.

order to visualize a well defined, circular, cross-sectional view of the artery. Next, identify the axillary vein, which should be located just caudal to the artery. Once both the axillary artery and vein have been identified, look for the three *hyperechoic* cords typically located at approximately 3-o'clock, 6-o'clock, and 9-o'clock around the axillary artery (Figure 7.1, Figure 7.5). The posterior cord is usually located near the 6-o'clock position, posterior to the axillary artery. The posterior cord may be obscured by the acoustic enhancement artifact from the axillary artery. The medial or lateral cords can typically be located near either the 3-o'clock or 9-o'clock position, depending on which side of the patient is being scanned. The lateral cord is positioned cephalad to the axillary artery, whereas the medial cord is positioned caudad to the artery and is typically located between the axillary artery and vein. Once these structures have been identified, we advise to complete scanning in the vicinity near the cords to identify the proximity of the hyperechoic rib and, therefore, pleura (Figure 7.9). Also, look in the vicinity where the

needle will be traveling (from cephalad) to identify whether there are any significant vascular structures located along its potential path (Figure 7.10).

Additional considerations

When positioning the patient, the arm may also be abducted approximately 90 degrees, which may move the brachial plexus further away from the ribcage and, therefore, the lung. This positioning technique may be beneficial on very thin patients or for patients who have a very close proximity of the brachial plexus to the ribcage on initial scan.

When performing the initial scan and having difficulty identifying the axillary vein, it may be due to the operator pressing too hard on the skin with the ultrasound probe. This may collapse the axillary vein and distort the overall anatomy.

When uncertain as to whether a hypoechoic structure is vasculature, use either the color-flow (Figure 7.11) and/or pulse-wave Doppler (Figure 7.12) functions on the ultrasound machine to help identify the structure in question.

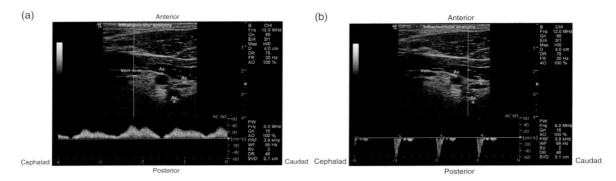

Figure 7.12 (a) and (b) Same infraclavicular region using pulse-wave Doppler to identify anomalous vascular structures.

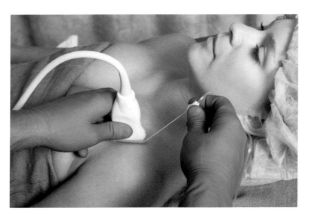

Figure 7.13 Ultrasound and in-plane needle position for performance of an infraclavicular brachial plexus block.

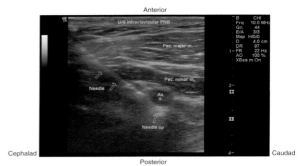

Figure 7.14 Ideal initial needle placement adjacent to posterior cord for infraclavicular brachial plexus block.

Needle insertion

Once an adequate image has been obtained and it has been deemed safe to perform the block, a skin wheal is raised with local anesthetic at the cephalad end of the ultrasound probe. A blunt-tipped needle is placed through the wheal and advanced *in plane* (IP) with the ultrasound beam in a cephalad to caudad direction, posteriorly towards the brachial plexus (Figure 7.13). Look for the needle or movement in the upper corner (anterior–cephalad) of the screen. Once the needle is under the transducer, it should become visible as a hyperechoic line. Do not blindly advance the needle. If the needle is not initially visible, stop and look at your hands to make sure that the needle is passing straight in the beam of the ultrasound probe. If it appears as though it should be but the needle remains not visible on the screen, you may need to make very small tilting or rotating movements with the probe to bring the

needle into view. The initial image of your target structures should change very minimally, if at all. If the original scan has changed significantly in order to locate the needle, remove the needle and begin from the initial scanning step. The path of the needle should be aimed just posterior to the axillary artery. The ideal initial needle tip placement before injection should be posterior to the axillary artery, just next to the posterior cord (Figure 7.14). Special care should be taken to avoid contacting the cords of the brachial plexus in order to minimize the potential for nerve damage.

Additional considerations

The most important part of the needle to keep in constant visualization is the needle tip. If the tip is not constantly visualized, it is difficult to be certain as to where it is located and what structures it may be penetrating. The only part of the needle that can be visualized is the part that is traveling through the narrow ultrasound beam.

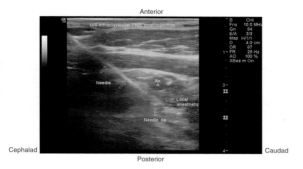

Figure 7.15 Appropriate local anesthetic spread around axillary artery for infraclavicular brachial plexus block.

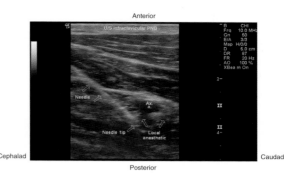

Figure 7.16 Appropriate local anesthetic spread for infraclavicular brachial plexus block *with* compression of the axillary artery.

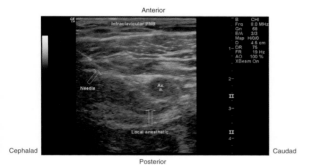

Figure 7.17 Injection at posterior cord with contained spread of local anesthetic to lateral and posterior cord.

Local anesthetic injection and needle repositioning

Due to the separation of the cords of the brachial plexus by the axillary artery, adequate spread of local anesthetic to all three cords may require multiple passes of the block needle. With the needle tip positioned adjacent to the posterior cord, injection of the local anesthetic can begin. Frequent confirmation of negative aspiration initially and after approximately every 3 to 5 ml of injection should be performed. Stopping injection to aspirate every 3 to 5 ml can help slow down the speed of injection, which can potentially decrease the pressure of injection. If there is high resistance to injection, stop and reposition the needle. Pay special attention to the spread of the local anesthetic, which will appear as an expanding hypoechoic region. It should be in a well contained space, spreading both cephalad and caudad around the axillary artery in a crescent shape towards the lateral and medial cords (Figure 7.15). This often causes compression of the axillary artery

and, in fact, this finding is consistent with a higher success rate of the block (Figure 7.16). If the local anesthetic spreads from the posterior cord to surround both the medial and lateral cords, then the needle tip need not be repositioned throughout injection as long as no intravascular or intraneural injection is suspected. If the local anesthetic is not spreading as described, the needle should be repositioned (Figure 7.17). If the spread of the local anesthetic does not properly surround the lateral cord, the needle should be slowly pulled back along the original entry path until the tip of the needle is located adjacent to the lateral cord. After negative aspiration of heme, inject more local anesthetic in 3- to 5-ml increments, continuing to pay special attention to visualizing the spread of the local anesthetic within the appropriate fascial plane. If the local anesthetic does not properly surround the medial cord, the needle can be pulled back along its original path slightly more, to position the needle tip between the lateral cord and the fascia of the pectoralis minor. Injection of local anesthetic here may reach the medial cord by spreading superficial to the axillary artery. Alternatively, the needle can be pulled back even more, superficial to the fascia of the pectoralis minor, then flatten the angle of the needle (lower the hub of the needle toward the patient) and advance at a more obtuse angle. This will have the needle pass just anterior/superficial to the axillary artery, then through the fascia of the pectoralis minor, so that the tip of the needle is located adjacent to the medial cord (Figure 7.18). Take special care to avoid puncture of the axillary vein. After negative aspiration of heme, the remaining local anesthetic volume is injected in 3- to 5-ml increments, again paying special attention to visualizing the spread of the local anesthetic within the appropriate fascial plane. Now the infraclavicular brachial plexus block is complete. With enough experience, this block should be performed with just one to two needle passes.

Additional considerations

A negative aspiration does not rule out an intravascular injection.

Remain alert to the possibility of intravascular injection if the spread of local anesthetic is not seen, as this may indicate that the local anesthetic is being deposited into a vessel and not perineurally.

Stopping injection after every 3 to 5 ml in order to reconfirm negative aspiration of blood can help slow down the speed of injection, which can potentially decrease the pressure of injection.

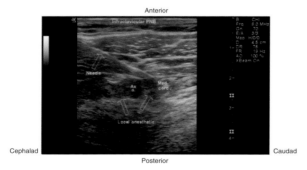

Figure 7.18 Needle repositioned with tip at medial cord.

Block of the intercostobrachial nerve

Block of the intercostobrachial nerve occurs high in the axilla. First, the patient's arm is abducted approximately 90 degrees and a sterile preparation is applied to the upper arm. Next, local anesthetic in a 10-ml syringe is injected with a 3-cm, 25-gage needle subcutaneously, forming a linear wheal along the axillary crease from the anterior head of the deltoid muscle to the long head of the triceps muscle (Figure 7.19).

Additional considerations

We recommend performing the intercostobrachial nerve block *after* the brachial plexus block, since it may be painful for some patients to abduct their arm.

If one will be using the infraclavicular block as the primary anesthetic for any procedure in which an upper arm tourniquet is to be used, it may be beneficial to supplement with an intercostobrachial nerve block. This makes the discomfort from the squeeze of the tourniquet more tolerable to the patient.

Authors' clinical practice

- *Dosing regimen:* to maximize block duration for postoperative pain control while decreasing onset time for surgical anesthesia, we typically use 30 to 40 ml of 0.75% ropivacaine for our infraclavicular nerve blocks. The volume and dose of anesthetic used will be influenced by the patient, the patient's history and relevant comorbid conditions, and the spread of the local anesthetic.

- Use of shorter acting agents, such as mepivacaine or lidocaine, in place of ropivacaine may be more

(a) (b)

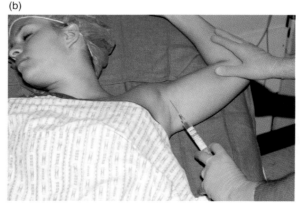

Figure 7.19 (a) and (b) Performance of intercostobrachial nerve block.

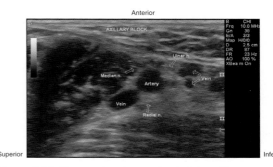

Figure 8.11 Ultrasound anatomy at level of the axilla.

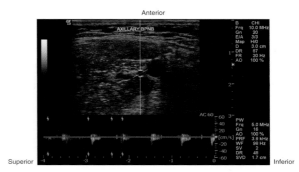

Figure 8.13 Doppler imaging to aid in detection of vascular structures in the axilla.

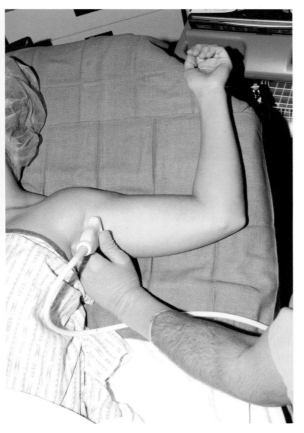

Figure 8.10 Ultrasound examination of patient prior to axillary brachial plexus block.

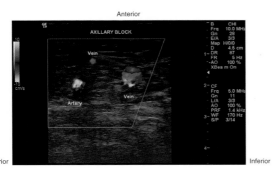

Figure 8.12 Color-flow imaging to aid in detection of vascular structures in the axilla.

placed in contact with the patient's skin in order to produce an adequate transverse image of the axilla. Initially, enough pressure should be used to keep the entire probe on the patient, but not so much pressure that superficial veins will collapse. Once oriented, varying the amount of pressure on the probe can actually be helpful in identifying venous structures that may not be readily apparent at first. Utilization of color-flow or Doppler imaging can also be helpful in identifying the presence of blood vessels to be avoided in the block area (Figures 8.11, 8.12, and 8.13).

The nerves in the axilla tend to have mixed echogenicity: hypoechoic centers (fascicles) are surrounded by hyperechoic rings (connective tissue). Cut in cross-section, the nerves usually have a rounded appearance as they appear around hypoechoic blood vessels.

Needle insertion

The best approach for block needle placement is one that minimizes the number of needle passes to each target while best avoiding vascular obstacles. The goal is to cover the necessary nerve distributions with as few needle passes as possible.

Additional considerations

For many, the initial nerve targeted for this block is the radial nerve as it tends to be the deepest.

73

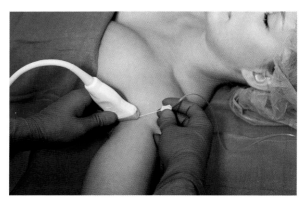

Figure 8.14 In-plane needle placement during brachial plexus block via an axillary approach.

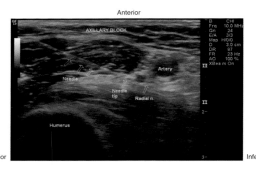

Figure 8.15 In-plane needle approach to the radial nerve in the axilla.

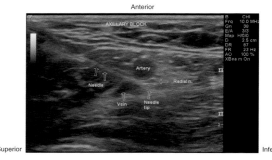

Figure 8.16 Targeting the radial nerve; note the proximity of a large vein to the target nerve.

The more superficial nerves are then covered by witnessing spread of the local anesthetic toward them, or by redirection of the needle.

A local skin wheal is made at the superior (cephalad) portion of the probe. A blunt-tipped needle is placed through the wheal and advanced *in-plane* (IP) with the ultrasound beam, in a cephalad to caudad direction posteriorly towards the brachial plexus (Figures 8.14 and 8.15). Look for the needle in the upper corner of the ultrasound screen near the screen indicator. Once the needle is under the transducer, it should become visible as a hyperechoic line. The target structures in this area will be superficial, typically <1 to 2 cm deep.

Do not blindly advance the needle. If the needle is not initially visible, stop and look at your hands to make sure that your needle is passing straight in the beam of the ultrasound probe. If it appears as though it should be, but the needle is still not clearly visible on the screen, you may need to make very

small tilting or rotating movements with the probe to bring the needle into view. The initial image of your target structures should change minimally, if at all. If the original scan has changed significantly in order to locate the needle, then remove the needle and begin again.

Depending on the patient's anatomy, all nerves around the artery can usually be blocked from this needle position as long as venous structures/obstacles permit.

Additional considerations

Remember that with an *in-plane* needle approach the only part of the needle that is visualized is the part traveling within the small ultrasound beam. This may or may not include the needle tip if the entire needle is not visualized. An effort should therefore be made to keep the *entire shaft* of the needle within the ultrasound beam to maintain an awareness of tip location.

Local anesthetic injection and needle repositioning

With an awareness of vascular structures around the targeted nerves, additional pressure can be applied to help collapse small veins that might be in the needle's projected pathway. Local anesthetic injection is undertaken once the needle tip appears to be in a safe position adjacent to the target nerve (Figures 8.16–8.21). The injection should be performed in 3- to 5-ml increments with aspirations attempted between injections to further ensure the needle tip remains extra vascular. With ultrasound, anesthetic spread should *always* be observed with each injection. Failure to do so

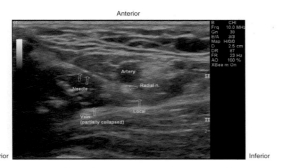

Figure 8.17 Local anesthetic injection in proximity to the radial nerve.

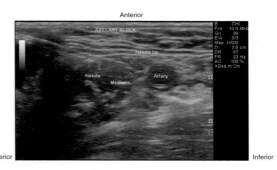

Figure 8.18 Targeting the median nerve.

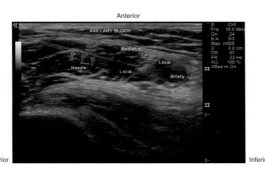

Figure 8.19 Local anesthetic injection in proximity to the median nerve.

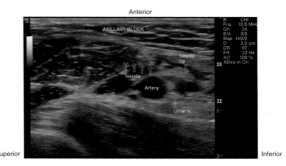

Figure 8.20 Targeting the ulnar nerve.

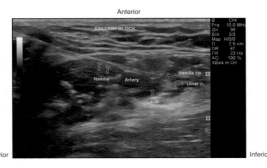

Figure 8.21 Local anesthetic injection in proximity to the ulnar nerve.

should prompt the operator to stop the injection immediately, regardless of a prior negative aspiration.

Additionally, pay attention to the amount of resistance encountered with injection. Stop injecting if an increased or unusually high injection pressure is noted as this can be a sign that the needle tip is in an undesirable location, and perhaps intraneural.

Additional considerations

Be aware of the nerve distribution that needs to be blocked in order to perform a successful anesthetic. It may not be necessary to block the entire plexus to provide anesthesia or analgesia for the surgical area. Knowing the anatomy and nerve supply allows one to concentrate the local anesthetic deposition at points that will have the most benefit.

Keep in mind that a successful ultrasound-guided block performed at the axilla typically requires anesthetic be deposited around the nerves themselves, not circumferentially around the artery. Due to anatomic variation, simply surrounding the artery with anesthetic may lead to partial failure of the block as some nerves (e.g., the radial nerve) may lie away from the vessel.

When injection is undertaken, the needle tip does not have to be positioned in contact with the nerve to block the nerve. In fact, doing so can risk injury. What is important is witnessing the *spread* of local anesthetic around nerves requiring blockade, and this can sometimes be achieved with few needle reposition movements. The spread of the local anesthetic will appear as an expanding hypoechoic region in a well contained space.

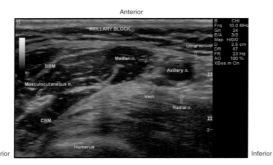

Figure 8.22 Identifying the musculocutaneous nerve (arrow) in the axilla. BBM = biceps brachii muscle, CBM = coracobrachialis muscle.

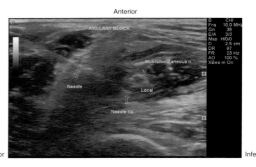

Figure 8.23 Needle insertion and anesthetic injection: axillary musculocutaneous nerve block.

If the first needle pass does not yield adequate spread around a particular nerve, the needle should be repositioned. Often more than one needle pass may be necessary to carefully surround the target nerve. From 30 to 35 ml of anesthetic is typically used to block the three nerves around the axillary artery.

Additional considerations

A negative aspiration does not rule out an intravascular injection. Pressure placed on the transducer to collapse venous structures can lead to a false negative aspiration when the needle tip is actually positioned in a vein.

Remain alert to the possibility of intravascular injection if the spread of local anesthetic is not seen, as this may indicate that the local anesthetic is being deposited into a vessel.

Block of the musculocutaneous nerve

The musculocutaneous nerve must be identified and anesthetized separately with the axillary block approach. In addition to providing motor innervation for elbow flexion and supination of the wrist, the terminal extension of the musculocutaneous nerve provides cutaneous innervation to the lateral forearm. The *lateral antebrachial cutaneous nerve (lateral cutaneous nerve of the forearm)* is the terminal extension of the musculocutaneous nerve, emerging near the elbow and extending along the lateral forearm to the wrist. Procedures of the antecubital fossa, forearm, and wrist usually require blockade of the musculocutaneous nerve.

On ultrasound, the musculocutaneous nerve in the axilla can appear in different shapes (round, oval, teardrop, or flattened) and with mixed echogenicity. The nerve becomes sandwiched between the biceps brachii and coracobrachialis muscles superior to the axillary artery in the 7- to 10-o'clock position (Figure 8.22).

The needle insertion site is usually kept the same as that for blockade of the other axillary brachial plexus nerves but with steeper angling of the block needle. Five to 10 ml of local anesthetic are typically enough to surround the nerve completely (Figure 8.23).

Additional considerations

If difficulty is encountered in identifying the musculocutaneous nerve, proximal or distal movement of the probe from the starting point can sometimes help bring the nerve into view. When located, the nerve can then be followed back to the position desired to place the block.

Block of the intercostobrachial nerve

Block of the intercostobrachial nerve occurs high in the axilla. Keeping the patient's arm comfortably abducted (as when performing an axillary block approach), a sterile preparation solution is applied to the upper arm. Approximately 10 ml of local anesthetic is injected with a 3-cm, 25-gage needle subcutaneously, forming a linear wheal along the axillary crease from the anterior head of the deltoid muscle to the long head of the triceps muscle (Figure 8.24a and b). (See also Chapter 9: Additional upper extremity peripheral nerve blocks).

Authors' clinical practice

- *Dosing regimen*: to maximize block duration for postoperative pain control while decreasing onset time for surgical anesthesia, we typically use a total of 30 to 40 ml of 0.75% ropivacaine for blocking the brachial plexus nerves in the axilla. Approximately 10 ml of local anesthetic is used per nerve. The volume and dose of anesthetic is influenced by the patient, his/her

(a)

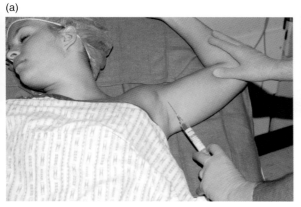

(b)

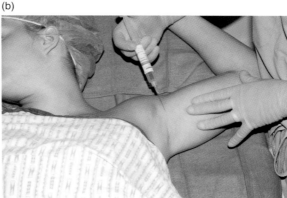

Figure 8.24 (a) and (b) Intercostobrachial nerve field block.

history, relevant comorbid conditions, and the spread of local anesthetic.

- For cases in which extended postoperative analgesia will not be necessary, mepivacaine with or without epinephrine is often substituted in 20- to 40-ml volumes.
- Some advantages to use of the ultrasound-guided axillary block approach include:
  - superficial nature of the target structures and ease of image acquisition
  - ease of needle identification given shallow angling during in-plane needle approach
  - probably greatly reduces, or eliminates, the risk of pneumothorax and phrenic nerve involvement
  - is performed at an easily compressible site should vascular injury occur.
- Some disadvantages to use of the ultrasound-guided axillary block approach include:
  - placement of anesthetic in a highly vascular area where multiple needle passes to each nerve are often required
  - the musculocutaneous nerve must be identified away from the axillary artery and blocked separately

- some patients may complain of axillary discomfort following block placement in this highly sensitive area
- abducting the extremity to be blocked may be difficult for some patients depending on the clinical situation (e.g., fracture, casted extremity, etc.)
- In our practice, the infraclavicular block is often substituted for the axillary block approach. However, we find use of the axillary block approach, especially for cases of the hand and wrist, to be safe, convenient, and effective when carefully performed under ultrasound guidance.

Suggested reading

Chan V W, Perlas A, McCartney C J, *et al.* (2007). Ultrasound guidance improves success rate of axillary brachial plexus block. *Can J Anaesth*, **54**(3):176–82.

Neal J M, Gerancher J C, Hebl J R, *et al.* (2009). Upper extremity regional anesthesia: essentials of our current understanding, 2008. *Reg Anesth Pain Med*, **34**(2):134–70.

Retzl G, Kapral S, Greher M, Mauritz W (2001). Ultrasonographic findings in the axillary part of the brachial plexus. *Anesth Analg*, **92**(5):1271–5.

Additional upper extremity peripheral nerve blocks

Superficial Cervical Plexus Block

Anatomy

The cervical plexus is formed from the anterior rami of C2 to C4. The fibers from C1 may form a loop with some fibers of C2. The cervical plexus lies beneath the sternocleidomastoid and contains both deep and superficial portions. The superficial portion emerges from the lateral border of the sternocleidomastoid. The superficial cervical plexus provides sensation to much of the skin overlying the shoulder, neck, and upper thorax. The branches of the superficial cervical plexus are: (1) the *lesser occipital nerve*, (2) the *great auricular nerve*, (3) the *transverse cervical nerves*, and (4) the *supraclavicular nerves (lateral, middle, and medial)* (Figure 9.2). The *supraclavicular nerves* are responsible for sensation over much of the shoulder and upper thorax (Figure 9.1).

Equipment

- 10-ml syringe
- 1½-inch, 25-gage needle
- Sterile gloves
- Sterile skin preparation
- Sterile skin marker

Technique

The block of the superficial cervical plexus is carried out at the lateral border of the sternocleidomastoid. The lateral border of the clavicular head of the sternocleidomastoid is traced from the mastoid to its attachment on the clavicle, and divided in half. Half of the volume of local anesthetic is fanned superficially along the lateral border of the sternocleidomastoid, superior to the midpoint of the sternocleidomastoid, and the other half is fanned superficially along the lateral border of the sternocleidomastoid, inferior to

Figure 9.1 Sensory nerve distribution to upper extremity.

Posterior Arm

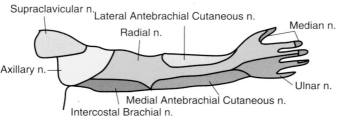

Anterior Arm

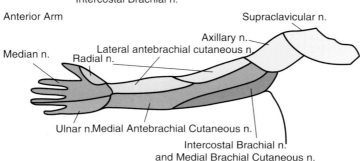

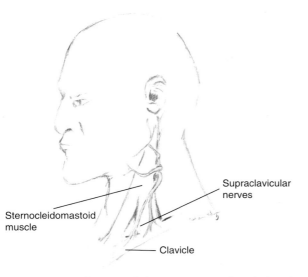

Figure 9.2 Superficial cervical plexus as it emerges from the lateral border of the sternal head of the sternocleidomastoid.

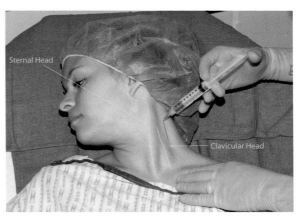

Figure 9.3 Local anesthetic being deposited along the lateral border of the clavicular head of the sternocleidomastoid. Notice the prominent sternal head of the sternocleidomastoid and a less prominent clavicular head.

the midpoint (Figures 9.2 and 9.3). This is a field block and is not a cutaneous nerve block, nor is it a deep cervical plexus nerve block. The local anesthetic should be deposited at the depth of the sternocleidomastoid.

Complications

Subarachnoid injection, epidural injection, and phrenic nerve block can be avoided by making sure the injection is at the depth of the sternocleidomastoid and not deeper. To avoid the possibility of a pneumothorax, do not carry out the inferior portion of the injection too inferiorly as the lung may extend above the clavicle in some patients.

Authors' clinical practice

- We typically use 5 to 10 ml of 0.5% or 0.75% ropivacaine for this block.
- Local anesthetic injected during an interscalene brachial plexus block may spread proximally to the C2–C4 nerve roots and block the superficial cervical plexus. The proximal spread from an interscalene block to the C2–C4 nerve roots may regress early and lead to early resolution of the superficial cervical plexus block. Therefore, we may perform a superficial cervical plexus block when the surgical procedure involves the clavicle or an open shoulder procedure.
- Patients undergoing open or arthroscopic shoulder surgery following a successful interscalene block may experience cutaneous pain in the anterior or posterior shoulder from the open incision or an anterior/posterior port hole in the distribution of the superficial cervical plexus. You may consider a separate block of the superficial cervical plexus in these patients.
- If a supraclavicular brachial plexus block is used for shoulder surgery in place of an interscalene brachial plexus block, then supplementation with a suprascapular nerve block along with a superficial cervical plexus block is recommended.

Suprascapular nerve block
Anatomy

The **suprascapular nerve** is formed from the upper trunk of the brachial plexus and contains fibers from C5 and C6. The nerve travels posteriorly through the suprascapular notch as it passes between the supraspinatus and infraspinatus muscles, providing motor innervation to these muscles. The supraclavicular nerve provides sensory innervation to the shoulder capsule, glenohumeral joint, and the acromioclavicular joint.

Equipment

- 10-ml syringe
- 1½-inch, 25-gage needle
- Sterile gloves
- Sterile skin preparation
- Sterile skin marker

79

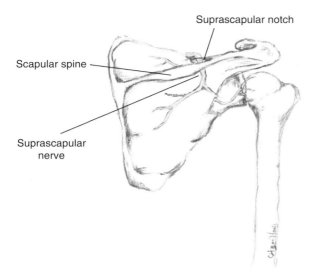

Figure 9.4 Suprascapular nerve as it passes through the scapular notch.

Technique

This block is best carried out with the patient in the sitting position, with the arm internally rotated. Identify the spine of the scapula and its midpoint. The needle is inserted in a parasagittal plane and directed caudal until the spine of the scapula is encountered. The local anesthetic is "fanned" along the superior aspect of the spine of the scapula (Figures 9.4 and 9.5).

Complications

A pneumothorax may result if this block is performed incorrectly. To decrease the chance of pneumothorax, maintain a caudal direction of the needle and avoid anterior direction. Internal rotation of the arm moves the scapula laterally and away from the lung, which may decrease the risk of a pneumothorax.

Authors' clinical practice

- We use 5 to 10 ml of 0.75% ropivacaine to perform this block. If a supraclavicular brachial plexus block is used for shoulder surgery in place of an interscalene brachial plexus block, then supplementation with a suprascapular nerve block is recommended.
- A suprascapular nerve block along with a superficial cervical plexus block will provide analgesia for a patient undergoing shoulder surgery when an interscalene nerve block or supraclavicular nerve block is not possible or contraindicated.

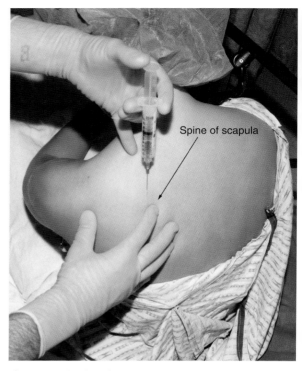

Figure 9.5 The shoulder is internally rotated and the needle is being directed in a cephalad to caudad direction.

Intercostobrachial

Anatomy

The intercostobrachial nerve arises primarily from the T2 intercostal nerve, with occasional supply from T1 or T3. Thus, it is not a component of the brachial plexus and is not anesthetized by a brachial plexus block. The intercostobrachial nerve provides cutaneous sensation in the axilla as well as the upper medial and posterior arm. The medial brachial cutaneous nerve and the medial antebrachial cutaneous nerve travel near the intercostobrachial nerve and all provide sensory innervation to the axilla, the upper medial and posterior arm, and the medial portion of the forearm (Figure 9.6).

Equipment

- 10-ml syringe
- 1½-inch, 25-gage needle
- Sterile gloves
- Sterile skin preparation
- Sterile skin marker

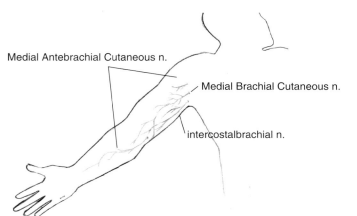

Medial Antebrachial Cutaneous n.

Medial Brachial Cutaneous n.

intercostalbrachial n.

Figure 9.6 Intercostobrachial nerve, medial brachial cutaneous nerve, and medial antebrachial cutaneous nerve.

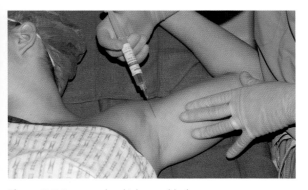

Figure 9.7 Intercostobrachial nerve block.

Technique

From 5 to 10 ml of local anesthetic is placed subcutaneously along the axillary crease from the anterior head of the deltoid muscle to the long head of the triceps muscle (Figure 9.7). Keep in mind that this is a cutaneous block.

Complications

Due to the superficial location of this block, there are no complications aside from bleeding and/or infection, which are potential complications of all nerve blocks.

Authors' clinical practice

- We use 5 to 10 ml of 0.5% ropivacaine to perform this block.
- An intercostobrachial nerve block may be used to alleviate some of the cutaneous discomfort associated with a tourniquet. True tourniquet pain is complex and partially due to muscle ischemia and will not be alleviated by this cutaneous block. However, block of the cutaneous nerves may aid in the intraoperative management of the patient if a purely regional technique is used.
- We use this block as a supplement for any surgery involving the elbow or upper arm as the incision may extend into the area innervated by the intercostobrachial nerve. Field block of the intercostobrachial nerve will also provide coverage of the medial brachial cutaneous and medial antebrachial cutaneous nerves.

Suggested reading

Abram S. (1999). Central hyperalgesic effects of noxious stimulation associated with the use of tourniquets. *Reg Anesth Pain Med*, **24**(2):99–101.

Neal J M, Gerancher J C, Hebl J R, *et al.* (2009). Upper extremity regional anesthesia: essentials of our current understanding, 2008. *Reg Anesth*, **34**(2):134–70.

10 Lower extremity anatomy for regional anesthesia

The practice of regional anesthesia requires a sound understanding of anatomy. In the application of this knowledge, it is important to understand that although there are many consistencies in anatomy from one person to the next, there are also inconsistencies. Thorough knowledge and understanding of applied anatomy, as well as relative anatomy, will lay the groundwork for a successful practice of regional anesthesia. In this chapter, the basic anatomy for successful performance of regional anesthetic procedures for the lower extremity described later in this book will be introduced. In order to practice safe and successful lower extremity regional anesthesia, a fundamental understanding of the lumbar plexus and sacral plexus is necessary.

The lumbar plexus

The lumbar plexus (Figure 10.1) innervates much of the skin and subcutaneous tissue (dermatomes), muscle (myotomes), and bones (osteotomes) of the lower abdominal wall, pelvis, genitalia, and the medial and anterior aspects of the thigh. It primarily arises from the ventral rami of the L1 through L4 spinal nerves, with occasional contribution from the T12 and/or L5 segments as well. The plexus forms in the posterior abdominal wall anterior to the transverse processes of the vertebrae, deep within the psoas muscle. As it travels distally, the lumbar plexus quickly begins to give off branches to the surrounding musculature (psoas major/minor, iliacus, and quadratus lumborum muscles), and begins to divide into some of the terminal nerves as the *iliohypogastric* (L1, +/− T12), *ilioinguinal* (L1), and *genitofemoral nerves* (L1 and L2). The lumbar plexus then divides into an anterior division, from which the *obturator nerve* (L2 through L4) arises, and a posterior division, from which the *femoral* (L2 through L4) and *lateral femoral cutaneous nerves* (L2 and L3) arise.

- The *iliohypogastric nerve* is formed by fibers originating from the L1 (and sometimes T12) level. It travels laterally from the psoas major

muscle, and passes through the transverse abdominus muscle to the level of the pubic symphysis. It provides muscle innervation along its path and supplies cutaneous sensation to the skin over the inferior abdomen and anterior hip.

- The *ilioinguinal nerve* is formed by fibers originating from the L1 level. It travels along the abdominal wall and passes through the inguinal canal. It provides muscle innervation along its path and supplies cutaneous sensation to the medial aspect of the proximal thigh and the anterior portion of the scrotum or labia majora.

- The *genitofemoral nerve* is formed by fibers originating from the L1 and L2 levels. It travels

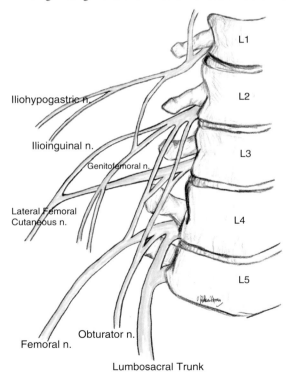

Figure 10.1 Organization of the lumbar plexus.

83

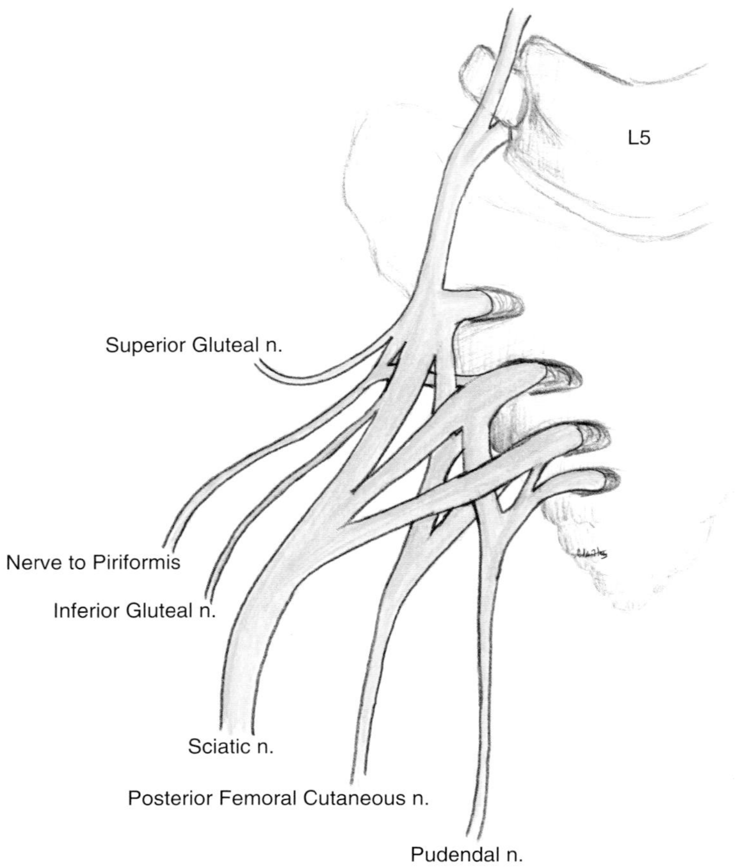

Figure 10.2 Organization of the sacral plexus.

L5

Superior Gluteal n.

Nerve to Piriformis

Inferior Gluteal n.

Sciatic n.

Posterior Femoral Cutaneous n.

Pudendal n.

along the abdominal wall and passes through the inguinal canal. While in the inguinal canal, it divides into a *femoral* branch, which pierces the abdominal wall to supply cutaneous sensation to the femoral triangle, then continues as the *genital* branch to provide innervation to the cremaster muscle and supply cutaneous sensation to the fascia and skin of the scrotum or labia majora.

- The *obturator nerve* is formed by fibers originating from the L2 through L4 levels. It travels medial to the psoas major muscle and passes through the obturator canal with the obturator artery and vein into the medial aspect of the thigh. Here it divides into an anterior and a posterior branch that continue to supply several of the muscles along the medial thigh primarily involved in adduction of the thigh, as well as flexion and extension of the thigh. The obturator nerve supplies cutaneous sensation to the medial

aspect of the thigh as the *medial femoral cutaneous nerves*, and provides sensation to the hip joint and the medial aspect of the knee joint.

- The *femoral nerve* is formed by fibers originating from the L2 through L4 levels. It travels lateral to the psoas major muscle and passes under the inguinal ligament with the femoral artery and vein, lateral to the vessels, into the anterior thigh. It provides muscle innervation along its path and, once in the thigh, divides into many branches to provide muscle innervation to many of the muscles of the anterior thigh including the rectus femoris, sartorius, and quadriceps muscles. The muscles that the femoral nerve innervates are involved in flexion and lateral rotation of the thigh, as well as extension of the leg with some flexion of the leg (sartorius muscle). It also supplies cutaneous sensation to the anterior thigh, as the *anterior femoral cutaneous nerves*, and the medial leg and ankle with variable extension into the

Table 10.1 Summary of lumbo-sacral plexus terminal nerve functions

Lumbo-sacral plexus terminal branch	Cutaneous sensation	Joint sensation	Motor action
Iliohypogastric nerve (L1, +/−T12)	Inferior abdomen Anterior hip	None	Abdominal muscles (transverse abdominus and obliques)
Ilioinguinal nerve (L1)	Medial, proximal thigh Anterior scrotum/labia majora	None	Abdominal muscles (transverse abdominus and obliques)
Genitofemoral nerve (L1, L2)	Over femoral triangle Fascia and skin of scrotum/labia majora	None	Elevation of scrotum (cremaster muscle)
Obturator nerve (L2–L4)	Medial aspect of thigh Medial aspect of knee	Anteromedial hip Flexion of thigh	Adduction of thigh Extension of thigh
Femoral nerve (L2–L4)	Anterior thigh Medial leg and ankle, +/− medial foot	Anterior hip Knee	Flexion and lateral rotation of thigh Extension of leg Flexion of leg
Lateral femoral cutaneous nerve (L2, L3)	Lateral thigh	None	None
Pudendal nerve (S2–S4)	Much of external genitalia	None	Muscles of perineum
Posterior cutaneous nerve of thigh (S1–S3)	Posterior thigh Posterior leg	None	None
Sciatic nerve (L4–S3)	See below for terminal branches	Posterior and posteromedial hip Posterior knee Ankle Foot	Flexion of thigh Adduction of thigh Flexion of leg See below for terminal branches
Superficial peroneal nerve (L4–S2)	Lateral leg Dorsal foot	None	Eversion of foot Plantarflexion of foot
Deep peroneal nerve (L4–S2)	Webspace between first and second toes	Ankle	Inversion of foot Dorsiflexion of foot Extension of toes
Tibial nerve (L4–S3)	Plantar surface of foot	Ankle Foot	Flexion of leg Plantarflexion of foot Flexion of toes Adduction and abduction of toes
Sural nerve (S1)	Lateral foot and fifth toe	Lateral ankle	None

medial foot as the *saphenous nerve*. It also provides sensation to the hip and knee joints.

- The *lateral femoral cutaneous nerve* is formed by fibers originating from the L2 and L3 levels. It travels laterally from the psoas major muscle, along the iliacus muscle, towards the anterior superior iliac spine (ASIS) and passes under the lateral portion of the inguinal ligament. Here it supplies cutaneous sensation along the lateral aspect of the thigh down to the knee.

The sacral plexus

The sacral plexus (Figure 10.2) innervates much of the skin and subcutaneous tissue (dermatomes), muscle (myotomes), and bones (osteotomes) of the

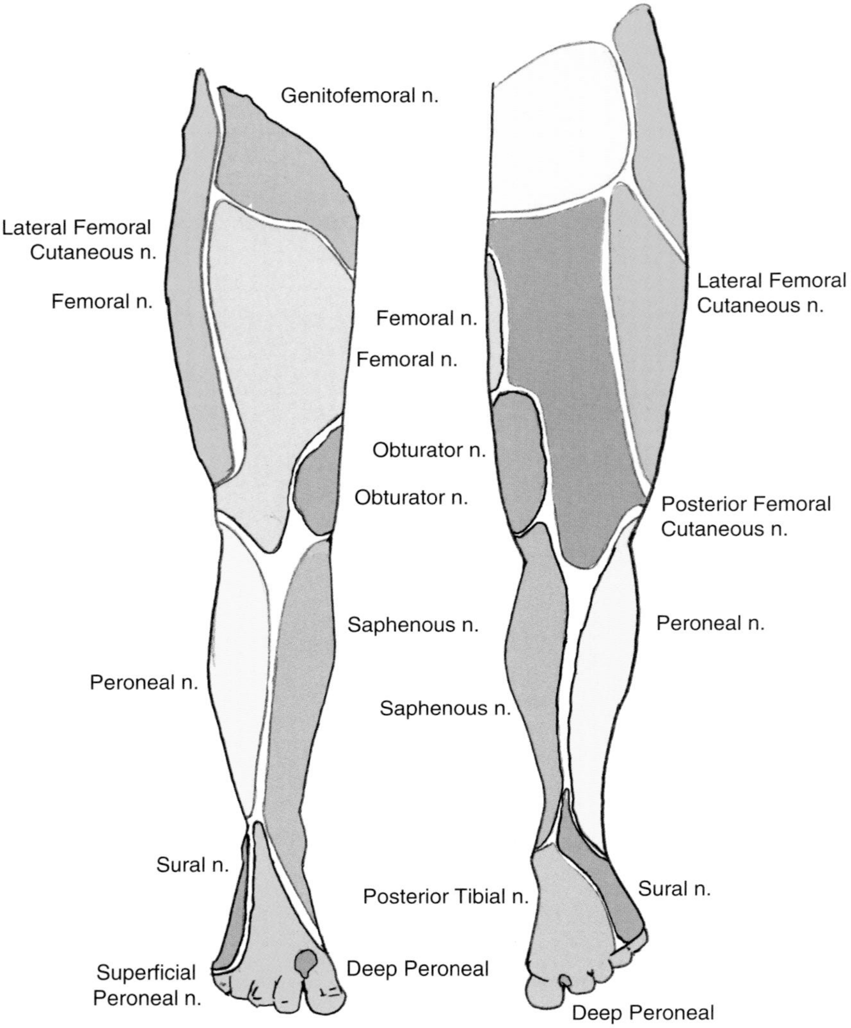

Figure 10.3 Sensory nerve distribution to the lower extremity.

gluteal, pelvic, posterior thigh, and much of the leg regions. It arises from the ventral rami of the L4 through S4 spinal nerves, as the lumbosacral trunk (L4 and L5) descends along the medial border of the psoas major muscle to join the sacral plexus at the S1 level. The plexus travels near the posterior wall of the pelvis towards the greater sciatic foramen. Along its course, the sacral plexus gives off several branches to the surrounding musculature (gluteus maximus/minimus, quadratus femoris, obturator internus, piriformis, levator ani, and external anal sphincter muscles), as well as the *pudendal nerve* (S2 through S4), which provides innervation to the muscles of the perineum and supplies cutaneous sensation to much of the external genitalia, and the *posterior cutaneous nerve of the thigh* (S1 through S3), which supplies cutaneous sensation to the posterior aspect of the thigh and leg. The sacral plexus then continues as the *sciatic nerve* (L4 through S3), its main terminal nerve, through the greater sciatic foramen into the gluteal region.

The sciatic nerve is created by the combination of the *common peroneal nerve* (L4 through S2) with the *tibial nerve* (L4 through S3). Occasionally these nerves travel separately, side by side, from their origin off the sacral plexus. The sciatic nerve travels out of the posterior pelvis, through the greater sciatic foramen, into the gluteal region. Here, it passes lateral to the ischial tuberosity, in the fascial plane between the gluteus maximus (superficially) and obturator internus (deeply) muscles, as it enters the posterior thigh.

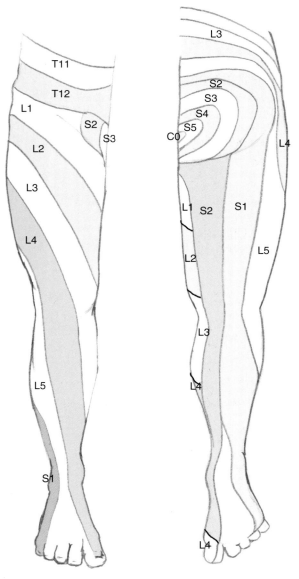

Figure 10.4 Lower extremity dermatomes.

Once in the thigh it travels posterior to the femur within the "sciatic groove" formed by the biceps femoris (laterally) and semitendinosus and semimembranosus (medially) muscles, toward the popliteal fossa. Along its path, the sciatic nerve innervates the adductor magnus, biceps femoris, semitendinosus, and semimebranosus muscles that aid in adduction and flexion of the thigh, as well as flexion of the knee. The sciatic nerve and its terminal branches provide sensation to the posterior hip and the posteromedial

aspect of the hip joint capsule, posterior knee and ankle joints, as well as all the joints in the foot. When the sciatic nerve enters the popliteal fossa, on the posterior aspect of the knee, it separates into the common peroneal and tibial nerves. Shortly after the bifurcation of the sciatic nerve into these two nerves, they each supply a branch that combine to form the *sural nerve*.

- The *common peroneal nerve* is formed by fibers originating from the L4 through S2 levels. It travels lateral from the bifurcation of the sciatic nerve, passing with the distal tendon of the biceps femoris muscle towards the fibula, where it divides into its *superficial* and *deep* branches.
- The *superficial peroneal nerve* travels distally in the lateral aspect of the leg, providing innervation to muscles involved in eversion and plantarflexion of the foot. Along this path, it supplies cutaneous sensation to the lateral aspect of the leg. It then crosses the ankle into the foot as several nerve fibers that supply cutaneous sensation to the dorsal aspect of the foot.
- The *deep peroneal nerve* dives deep into the anterior aspect of the leg and travels distally, providing innervation to muscles involved in inversion and dorsiflexion of the foot. It then crosses into the foot along the anterior aspect of the ankle, providing innervation to muscles in the foot involved in extension of the toes, and supplies cutaneous sensation to the web space between the first and second toes.
- The *tibial nerve* is formed by fibers originating from the L4 through S3 levels. It travels medial and deep from the bifurcation of the sciatic nerve, between the two heads of the gastrocnemius muscle, into the posterior aspect of the leg. The nerve travels distally, providing innervation to muscles involved in flexion of the leg and plantarflexion of the foot. It then crosses the ankle into the foot along the posterior to the medial malleolus, usually posterior to the posterior tibial artery, where it then provides innervation to muscles involved in adduction, abduction, and flexion of the toes, as well as supplying cutaneous sensation to the plantar surface of the foot.
- The *sural nerve* is a pure sensory nerve that is formed by a branch of the common peroneal nerve as the *lateral sural nerve*, and a branch of the tibial nerve as the *medial sural nerve*, which are primarily formed from fibers

87

originating from the S1 level. These nerves combine to form the sural nerve near the level of the knee, which then travels distally between the heads of the gastrocnemius muscles, and becomes subcutaneous just lateral to the Achilles tendon in the mid to lower leg. The sural nerve then crosses into the ankle in the space between the lateral malleolus and the Achilles tendon, superficial to the fascia covering the ligaments, tendons, and muscles at the ankle. Along its path this nerve supplies sensation to the Achilles tendon and lateral ankle joint, then terminates by supplying cutaneous sensation to the lateral aspect of the foot and fifth toe.

Table 10.1 provides a summary of lumbo-sacral plexus terminal nerve functions.

Figure 10.3 shows sensory nerve distribution to the lower extremity. Figure 10.4 shows the dermatomes of the lower extremity.

Suggested reading

Birnbaum K, Prescher A, Hepler S, Heller K-D. (1997). The sensory innervation of the hip joint: an anatomical study. *Surg Radiol Anat*, **19**(6):371–5.

Netter F H. (2006). *Atlas of Human Anatomy*, 4th edn. Philadelphia: Saunders Elsevier.

Rohen J W, Yokochi C, Lutjen-Drecoll E. (2002). *Color Atlas of Anatomy: A Photographic Study of the Human Body*, 5th edn. Philadelphia: Lippincott Williams & Wilkins.

Sauerland E K. (1999). *Grant's Dissector*, 12th edn. Philadelphia: Lippincott Williams & Wilkins.

Sciatic nerve block: proximal approaches

Introduction and specific anatomy

The sciatic nerve can be blocked using ultrasound from numerous proximal positions along its course into the thigh. Such approaches include the gluteal or transgluteal (i.e., Labat) approach, subgluteal or infragluteal approach, anterior sciatic approach, and the lateral proximal thigh approach.

This chapter will focus on two proximal ultrasound-guided sciatic nerve blocking techniques: the subgluteal approach and the anterior approach. The *subgluteal approach* to the sciatic nerve can be performed with relative ease compared to other proximal approaches. The *anterior sciatic approach* to the sciatic nerve, while technically more difficult, allows the patient to remain supine while the block is placed. Both approaches provide anesthesia of the lower extremity when used in combination with femoral nerve or lumbar plexus blocks.

The sciatic nerve and branches

The sciatic nerve, the largest peripheral nerve in the human body, is formed from ventral roots of the lumbosacral plexus (L4–S3) (Figure 11.1).

Once formed, the sciatic nerve leaves the pelvis by coursing distally through the greater sciatic foramen. The nerve travels under the piriformis muscle, and over the dorsal aspect of the ischial bone, passing midway between the greater trochanter of the femur (lateral) and the ischial tuberosity (medial) before entering the posterior proximal thigh (Figure 11.2). Midway between the ischial tuberosity and the greater trochanter, the nerve is sandwiched between the gluteus maximus muscle (posterior) and the quadratus femoris muscle (anterior). At this point, the sciatic nerve provides some motor innervation to external rotators of the hip and may give articular branches to posterior portions of the hip capsule.

As the nerve continues into the proximal thigh, it remains between the adductor muscles of the hip

(anterior) and the gluteus maximus muscle (posterior) (Figure 11.3) before coursing behind the long head of the biceps femoris muscle. The nerve remains posteriorly positioned, deep to the hamstring muscles, and as it travels through the thigh providing motor innervation to the adductor magnus muscle and the hamstring muscles.

> **Additional considerations**
>
> The skin of the posterior thigh is innervated by the posterior femoral cutaneous nerve (S1–S3). Blockade of this nerve usually occurs via diffusion of a large volume of local anesthetic placed at proximal positions around the sciatic nerve (infragluteal). Sparing of the posterior femoral cutaneous nerve, and thus the skin of the posterior thigh, can occur when subgluteal or anterior block approaches are undertaken, necessitating use of supplemental blockade in some patients.

Entering the popliteal space created by the hamstring and gastrocnemius muscles (semitendinosis muscle and semimembranosis muscle superomedially; biceps femoris long head muscle superolaterally; medial and lateral heads of the gastrocnemius muscle inferiorly), the sciatic nerve divides medially to form the tibial nerve, and laterally to form the common peroneal nerve. The point where this bifurcation occurs is variable but generally occurs around the distal 2/3 portion of the patient's thigh near the popliteal space (Figure 11.4).

The *tibial nerve* (L4–S3), the larger of the two sciatic divisions, travels through the popliteal space lateral and superficial to the popliteal artery and vein before coursing medially into the lower leg behind the gastrocnemius muscle at the base of the fossa (Figure 11.4). The nerve follows a surface line down the leg from the center of the popliteal space to the midway point of the medial malleolus and the calcaneal tendon. The tibial nerve is responsible for

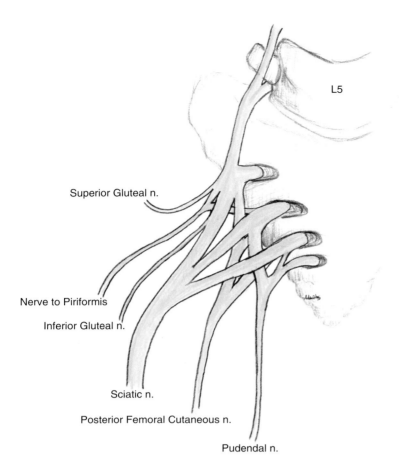

Figure 11.1 Organization of the sacral plexus.

L5

Superior Gluteal n.

Nerve to Piriformis

Inferior Gluteal n.

Sciatic n.

Posterior Femoral Cutaneous n.

Pudendal n.

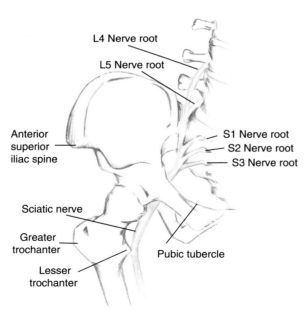

L4 Nerve root

L5 Nerve root

Anterior
superior
iliac spine

S1 Nerve root
S2 Nerve root
S3 Nerve root

Sciatic nerve

Greater
trochanter

Pubic tubercle

Lesser
trochanter

Figure 11.2 Sciatic nerve exiting the pelvis ASIS = anterior superior iliac spine; GT = greater trochanter; LT = Lesser trochanter; PT = pubic tubercle.

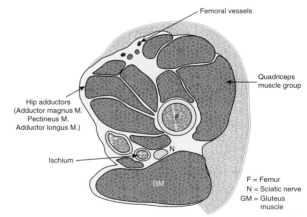

Femoral vessels

Quadriceps
muscle group

Hip adductors
(Adductor magnus M.
Pectineus M.
Adductor longus M.)

Ischium

F

N

GM

F = Femur
N = Sciatic nerve
GM = Gluteus
muscle

Figure 11.3 Cross-sectional image of the proximal thigh.

muscular innervation of the calf (popliteus, gastrocnemius, and soleus muscles) and flexor muscles of the foot (tibialis posterior, flexor digitorum longus, and flexor hallicus longis muscles), provides articular branches to the knee, and cutaneous innervation to most plantar portions of the foot and toes.

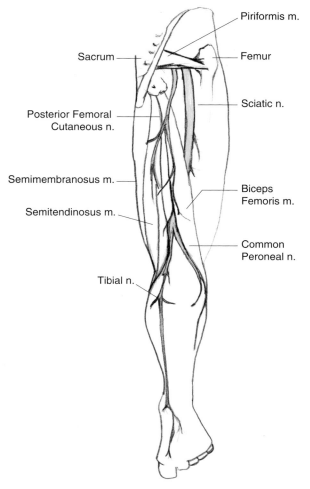

Sacrum

Posterior Femoral
Cutaneous n.

Semimembranosus m.

Semitendinosus m.

Tibial n.

Piriformis m.

Femur

Sciatic n.

Biceps
Femoris m.

Common
Peroneal n.

Figure 11.4 Posterior anatomy of the lower extremity with the sciatic nerve and its branches.

The *common peroneal nerve* (L4–S2) splits from the sciatic nerve and courses laterally across the popliteal space and around the fibular head and neck (Figure 11.4). The nerve travels distally behind the peroneus longus muscle along the lateral aspect of the lower leg only a short distance before dividing into the deep and superficial peroneal nerves.

The *deep peroneal nerve* descends deep to the muscles of the anterior leg along the interosseous membrane between the tibia and fibula. In the lower third of the leg, the deep peroneal nerve travels with the anterior tibial artery before crossing the ankle joint deep to the extensor retinaculum. The deep peroneal nerve supplies motor innervation to extensor muscles of the foot and ankle including the extensor hallucis longus, the extensor digitorum longus

and brevis, the tibialis anterior, and peroneus tertius muscles. The deep peroneal nerve provides sensory innervation to the ankle joint and the web space between the first and second toes (Figure 11.5).

The *superficial peroneal nerve* travels deep to the peroneal muscles, becoming superficial around the mid-portion of the lower leg. The nerve provides motor innervation to muscles of the lateral leg and ankle (peroneus longus and brevis muscles) and sensory innervation to the lateral leg and dorsum of the foot (Figure 11.5).

The *sural nerve* also provides cutaneous innervation to inferior portions of the lateral and posterior lower leg as well as the lateral aspect of the foot (Figure 11.5). The nerve typically forms along the lateral leg from cutaneous branches of both the tibial and common peroneal nerves (See also Chapter 10: Lower extremity anatomy for regional anesthesia). The sural nerve travels distally within deep fascia prior to becoming superficial and coursing around the posterior portion of the lateral malleolus.

Ultrasound anatomy
Subgluteal approach
Orienting structure (subgluteal approach): the greater trochanter (femur) and fascia

An appreciation of the musculoskeletal anatomy and fascial planes with this block approach will facilitate ultrasound imaging and target identification since a major vascular landmark is not present (Figure 11.6).

To image the pertinent structures for this regional technique, the patient is placed in the lateral position with the side to be blocked facing up. The hips and non-dependent knee are slightly flexed to increase clarity of the patient's surface anatomy. Depending on the size or body habitus of the patient, a linear or curved array probe may be used. The transducer is placed at the midpoint of an imaginary line connecting the patient's greater trochanter and ischial tuberosity on the side to be blocked. Note that the transducer should be placed perpendicular to the expected course of the sciatic nerve in order to produce a transverse image of the relevant anatomy (Figure 11.7).

The orienting structures for this block are the greater trochanter of the femur and the fascia separating the muscle bellies of the gluteus maximus muscle and quadratus femoris muscle.

An ultrasound image of this area appears essentially as two layers of muscle separated by fascia. The bony

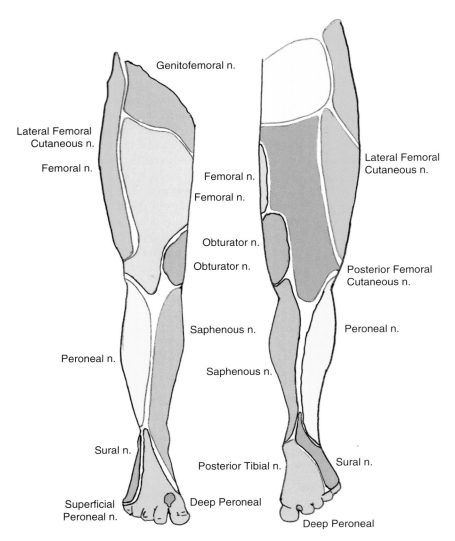

Figure 11.5 Sensory nerve distribution to the lower extremity.

Genitofemoral n.

Lateral Femoral
Cutaneous n.

Femoral n.

Femoral n.

Femoral n.

Lateral Femoral
Cutaneous n.

Obturator n.

Obturator n.

Posterior Femoral
Cutaneous n.

Saphenous n.

Peroneal n.

Peroneal n.

Saphenous n.

Sural n.

Sural n.

Posterior Tibial n.

Superficial
Peroneal n.

Deep Peroneal

Deep Peroneal

landmarks (greater trochanter and ischial tuberosity), on either side, appear to hold these muscle layers in place. Skin and subcutaneous tissue lie atop the most superficial layer: the gluteus maximus muscle. The thick gluteus maximus muscle has a striped texture typical of the mixed echogenicity of muscle. This muscle layer is separated from the next (the quadratus femoris muscle) by fascial planes that overlay the bodies of the muscle bellies. These fascial planes are hyperechoic and extend from the top of the greater trochanter to the ischial tuberosity when imaged in cross-section at this level. The sciatic nerve typically lies within this fascial plane, midway between the greater trochanter and the ischial tuberosity, and appears as a hyperechoic oval structure (Figure 11.6).

Additional considerations

If difficulty is initially encountered while trying to image the nerve at this point, adjusting the probe position by scanning proximally and distally along the center of the posterior thigh may be helpful. Often the nerve can be identified at a more distal position and then followed back to the location where the block will be placed.

Anterior sciatic approach
Orienting structure (anterior sciatic approach): the lesser trochanter (femur)

Imaging the sciatic nerve via a proximal, anterior app-roach is considered a more advanced ultrasound-guided

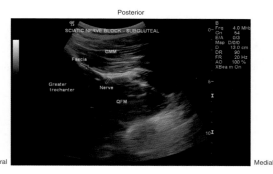

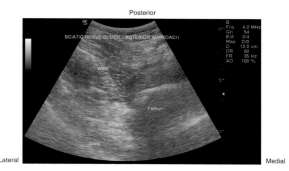

Figure 11.6 Sciatic nerve imaging via subgluteal approach. GMM = gluteus maximus muscle; QFM = quadratus femoris muscle.

Figure 11.8 Sciatic nerve imaging via anterior approach. GMM = gluteus maximus muscle; AMM = adductor magnus muscle.

Structures that are required to be identified	Structures that may be seen
Greater trochanter of femur	Quadratus femoris muscle
Fascial layer	Ischial tuberosity
Gluteus maximus muscle	

Structures that are required to be identified	Structures that may be seen
Lesser trochanter of femur	Femoral vessels
Fascia separating gluteus muscle from adductor muscles	
Addutor magnus muscle	
Gluteus maximus muscle	

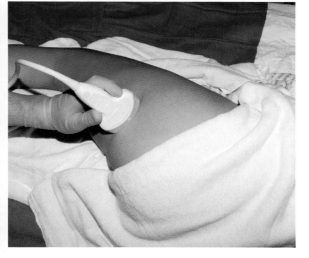

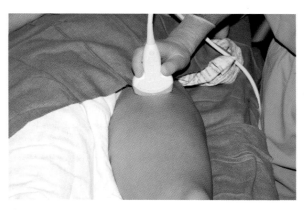

Figure 11.9 Probe positioning for a sciatic nerve block via an anterior approach.

Figure 11.7 Positioning the transducer for sciatic nerve block via the subgluteal approach.

regional technique (Figure 11.8). The patient is positioned supine with the ultrasound machine *at the foot of the bed* and the physician facing the machine. Using a low-frequency, curved array probe, the ultrasound transducer is positioned approximately 4 to 8 cm distal to the inguinal crease to start the examination (Figure 11.9). The probe should be moved proximally and distally, medially and laterally in order to confirm position of the orienting structure for this block approach: the lesser trochanter of the femur.

The hyperechoic edge of the lesser trochanter appears as a widening of the femur medially with an underlying hypoechoic bone shadow during scanning. A slight external rotation of the lower extremity and medial orientation of the probe can aid identification of the lesser trochanter during the initial assessment.

The hyperechoic sciatic nerve has a flattened appearance at this level and typically lies immediately

Table 11.1 Sample operative procedures for consideration of ultrasound-guided proximal sciatic nerve blocks

Procedure		Supplemental block[1]
Procedures of the distal leg	R	Femoral nerve/lumbar plexus or saphenous nerve +/− PFCN
Procedures of the mid leg	R	Femoral nerve/lumbar plexus or saphenous nerve +/− PFCN
Procedures of the proximal leg	R	Femoral nerve/lumbar plexus or saphenous nerve +/− PFCN
Procedures involving calcaneus or calcaneal (Achilles) tendon	R	Saphenous nerve or femoral nerve
Procedures of the ankle	M	Saphenous nerve or femoral nerve
Procedures involving multiple toes, midfoot or forefoot	M	Saphenous nerve

Note: R = recommended; M = maybe; NR = not recommended; PFCN = posterior femoral cutaneous nerve.
[1]Concomitant ipsilateral femoral nerve block provides complete anesthesia/analgesia of the lower extremity.

Table 11.2 Contraindications to ultrasound-guided proximal sciatic nerve blocks

Absolute contraindications	Relative contraindications
Patient refusal	Ipsilateral neuromuscular disease/damage
Infection over site of needle insertion	Contralateral neuromuscular disease/damage in ambulatory patient
Allergy to local anesthetics	Anticoagulation or bleeding disorder

Table 11.3 Side effects and complications associated with ultrasound-guided proximal sciatic nerve blocks

Side effects	Complications[1]
Motor blockade of foot and ankle for duration of local anesthetic effect	
Patient is at fall risk following block placement until block resolution	

Note: [1]Infection, nerve damage, local anesthetic toxicity, vascular injury, excessive bleeding, or hematoma are potential complications common to all nerve blocks.

adjacent to, or below, the lesser trochanter blending with the adjacent fascial layer (Figure 11.8).

The femoral artery and vein may be noted close to the skin above the femur. The vessels will appear relatively small compared with surrounding structures due to the use of a low-frequency, curved array transducer. Below the femoral vessels lie the adductor muscles of the hip.

The shape and depth (6 to 10 cm) of the nerve at this level can make identification a challenge on initial examination. A nerve stimulator is often helpful to confirm the nerve's position in this case.

Table 11.1 lists sample operative procedures for consideration of ultrasound-guided proximal sciatic nerve blocks.

Contraindications

Table 11.2 lists contraindications to ultrasound-guided proximal sciatic nerve blocks.

Side effects and complications

Table 11.3 shows some side effects and complications associated with ultasound-guided proximal sciatic nerve blocks.

Equipment

- Ultrasound machine with low-frequency (2 to 5 MHz) curved array transducer
- 8- or 10-cm, blunt-tipped needle (large or obese patients may require a 15-cm needle)
- Sterile cover for ultrasound probe
- Sterile ultrasound gel
- 2 to 3 ml of 1% lidocaine for local skin and subcutaneous infiltration
- Sterile gloves
- Appropriate local anesthetic and volume in 20-ml syringes
- Appropriate sedation, monitoring, and oxygen supply
- Illustrated in Figure 11.10

Technique
Technique summary

1. Monitors placed and patient appropriately sedated
2. Sterile preparation applied to procedural site
3. Clear Tegaderm™ applied to ultrasound probe

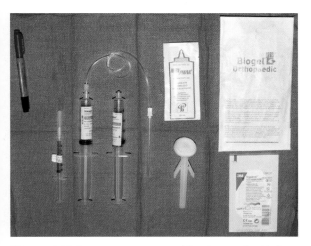

Figure 11.10 Equipment tray prepared for ultrasound-guided sciatic nerve block.

4. Perform systematic ultrasound scan to find optimal location for placement of nerve block
5. Skin wheal is raised
6. Insert block needle and guide toward target structures
7. Inject local anesthetic
8. Reposition needle as necessary to complete block

Subgluteal approach

Scanning

The patient is turned lateral to facilitate exposure of the area to be imaged, with the extremity to be blocked facing up. The hips and non-dependent knee are slightly flexed to increase clarity of the patient's surface anatomy. A pillow can be positioned between the patient's knees for added comfort.

For the subgluteal approach to the sciatic nerve, the ultrasound machine is placed *at the head of the bed*. We prefer to have the machine and the physician positioned on the side of the bed corresponding to the extremity being blocked, such that when the patient is turned lateral, his/her back is to the anesthesiologist performing the procedure (Figure 11.11). The clinician then faces the ultrasound machine at the head of the bed, scans with the hand closest to the patient, and guides the needle with the opposite hand. Thus for a *left* sciatic nerve block, the operator performs the ultrasound scan with the left hand while guiding the block needle with the right hand.

Following appropriate monitoring and sedation, the patient's greater trochanter and ischial tuberosity

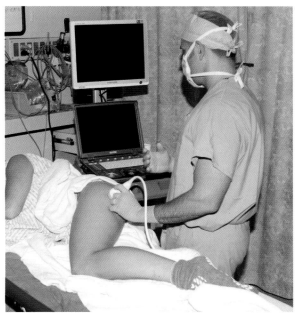

Figure 11.11 Transducer orientation for a sciatic nerve block via a subgluteal approach.

are first identified by palpation. The space between these bony landmarks is then prepared with a sterile preparation solution.

A low-frequency (5 MHz), curved array transducer, appropriately prepared with a sterile cover and conduction gel, is applied tranversly on the upper thigh at the midpoint along an imaginary line extending from the greater trochanter to the ischial tuberosity. Note that the position indicator on the transducer should be oriented to the patient's right and corresponds with the screen indicator typically set to the upper left-hand corner of the ultrasound image. This creates a transverse image of the structures, including the sciatic nerve, traversing the ultrasound beam below. Structures closest to the probe (skin/subcutaneous tissue) will appear at the top of the screen (Figure 11.12).

> **Additional considerations**
>
> Some patients may be small and/or thin enough that the subgluteal approach may be performed using higher frequency linear array transducers.

A fascial plane should be apparent below the gluteus maximus muscle, appearing to extend from the top of

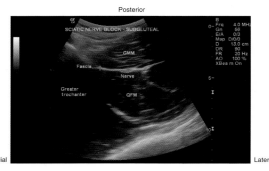

Figure 11.12 Scanning image prior to a sciatic nerve block via a subgluteal approach. GMM = gluteus maximus muscle; QFM = quadratus femoris muscle.

the greater trochanter toward the ischial tuberosity (see above: Ultrasound anatomy, subgluteal approach). The sciatic nerve is typically seen lying within this fascial plane, midway between the greater trochanter and the ischial tuberosity, and appears as a hyperechoic oval structure (Figure 11.12). At times the nerve may be flat enough to disappear, camouflaged within the fascial plane, though the nerve consistently remains below the gluteus maximus muscle midway between the bony structures.

Additional considerations

Use of a nerve stimulator to aid confirmation of the sciatic nerve's location can be useful when first learning this technique, or in cases where difficulty is encountered visualizing the nerve.

Note the depth setting on the ultrasound machine. The sciatic nerve will typically be imaged at a depth of 4 to 5 cm depending on the size of the patient. The depth setting on the machine should be set to allow imaging of the nerve and deeper structures (fascia and quadratus femoris muscle) that may be pertinent.

The gain and focal point should be adjusted to aid in identification of the hyperechoic fascial plane and sciatic nerve relative to the less echogenic muscle bellies above and below.

Additional considerations

Remember to have a systematic approach to scanning and probe movements that is consistent from one examination to the next.

To optimize the quality of the transverse image, subtle manipulations of the transducer are often

necessary. These manipulations may involve small changes in probe-tip direction (tilting, rotating, or sliding) and/or varying pressure applied to the probe during scanning.

Following the course of the nerve by scanning distally can also be a helpful way to confirm the nerve's position. Its course can then be followed back to a more proximal point.

Needle insertion

Having identified the sciatic nerve at the appropriate level, a skin wheal is placed along the lateral border (greater trochanter side) of the transducer with 1 to 2 ml of local anesthetic.

Needle positioning is undertaken with a blunt-tipped block needle introduced through the skin wheal using an in-plane approach (Figure 11.13). Look for the appearance of a hyperechoic line (needle) or tissue movement along the lateral edge of the ultrasound screen as the needle is advanced toward the fascial plane and sciatic nerve (Figure 11.14).

Additional considerations

An out-of-plane (OOP) approach to the nerve may also be used for this block. Benefits of an OOP approach may include easier needle manipulation and shorter needle distance to the target from the point of insertion. The disadvantage is greater difficulty in identification of needle-tip location.

Do not blindly advance the needle when using an in-plane approach. If you are having difficulty identifying the needle's location, stop and look at your hands to make sure that you are passing straight through the beam of the ultrasound probe. If your needle appears to be in-plane with the beam, but remains hidden on the screen, you may need to make very small tilting or rotating movements with the probe to bring the needle into view. The initial image of your target structures should change very minimally, if at all. If the original scan has changed significantly in order to locate the needle, then remove the needle and begin again.

Additional considerations

When difficulty in identifying the needle tip continues to be encountered, a *small* amount of local anesthetic (1 or 2 ml) may also be injected while

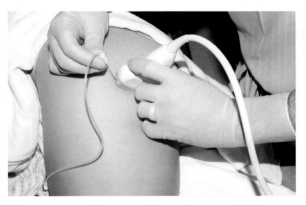

Figure 11.13 Needle insertion during placement of a left sciatic nerve block via a subgluteal approach.

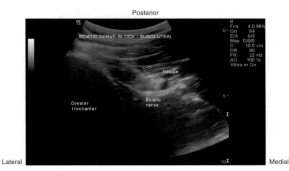

Figure 11.14 In-plane advancement of the needle during a subgluteal approach to the sciatic nerve.

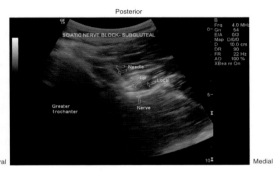

Figure 11.15 Local anesthetic injection during block of the sciatic nerve via a subgluteal approach.

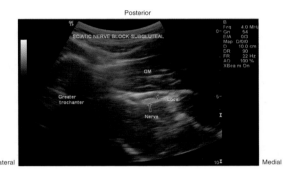

Figure 11.16 Local anesthetic surrounding the sciatic nerve following block via a subgluteal approach.

monitoring for tissue changes ("hydrolocation"). By changing the echogenicity of the surrounding tissue, hydrolocation may make needle-tip identification easier in some cases. If the injection is not observed on the ultrasound screen, however, it should be immediately stopped.

Though hydrolocation may be helpful at times, we do not advocate its routine use as a substitute for proper hand and needle positioning technique when performing an in-plane approach.

Local anesthetic injection and needle repositioning

The block needle should be placed in proximity to the nerve to pierce the surrounding fascia, without actually entering the nerve. The nerve itself will appear to be dissected away from the muscle as injection occurs ("hydrodissection"). During incremental injection, local anesthetic deposition should be visualized and monitored (Figure 11.15). A total of 20 to 40 ml of

local anesthetic can be injected depending on the patient, as well as anesthetic type and concentration used. When finished, a pocket of anesthetic should be adjacent to, or surrounding, the nerve (Figure 11.16).

Anterior sciatic approach

Scanning

The patient is positioned supine with the extremity to be blocked naturally extended and externally rotated at the hip. *The ultrasound machine is positioned at the foot of the bed.* This set up differs slightly from other block techniques described where the ultrasound machine is positioned at the head of the bed. Tissue depths of 6 to 10 cm and use of a low-frequency transducer may limit the clarity with which the sciatic nerve is imaged. Being able to see the patient's lower extremity as it is blocked may facilitate the concurrent use of a nerve stimulator if necessary.

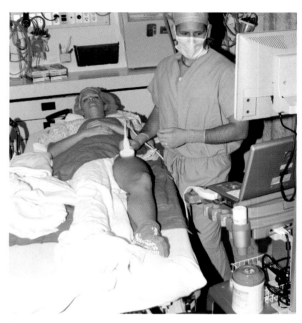

Figure 11.17 Scanning the proximal thigh prior to a sciatic nerve block via an anterior approach.

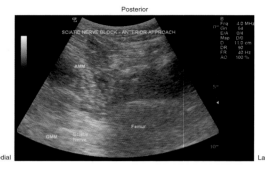

Figure 11.18 Sciatic nerve imaged via an anterior approach. AMM = adductor magnus muscle; GMM = gluteus maximus muscle.

Either physician hand may be used to perform the ultrasound scan. The key is making sure the scan and eventual needle placement can be done from a comfortable position. For example, if an in-plane, lateral approach to needle placement is used, it may be easiest to perform the scan with the hand closest to the patient while facing the ultrasound machine. Thus, to block the patient's left sciatic nerve, the physician's right hand performs the scan, while the block needle is placed from the lateral side of the patient's thigh with the left hand (Figures 11.17 and 11.19).

Following appropriate monitoring and sedation, the patient's inguinal crease and proximal thigh are disinfected with a sterile preparation solution. A low-frequency, curved array transducer is placed approximately 4 to 8 cm below the inguinal crease with the probe's position indicator to the patient's right. This creates a transverse image of the structures traversing the ultrasound beam.

Start by performing a systematic scan of the area looking for structures that will guide needle placement, specifically the femur and lesser trochanter.

Scan a short distance distally from the starting position. Make small changes medially and laterally as necessary to identify the hyperechoic bony edge of the femur and lesser trochanter. The lesser trochanter (laterally) should become apparent as a medial extension of the femur with proximal and/or distal position changes of the transducer. Note the thick gluteus maximus muscle deep to the lesser trochanter, and the anterior thigh muscles (adductors medially and quadriceps laterally) closest to the probe. The femoral vessels will appear relatively close to the surface and small relative to surrounding structures. The hyperechoic sciatic nerve has a flattened appearance at this level and typically lies immediately adjacent to, or below, the lesser trochanter in a layer of fascia separating the adductor muscles from the gluteus maximus muscle (Figure 11.18).

Additional considerations

Repositioning the probe medially can help to clarify the sciatic nerve's position when difficulty is encountered. Similarly, by making very subtle tilting movements in a cephalad or caudad direction, one can improve the angle of incidence at which the ultrasound beam is reflected, further optimizing the transverse image.

Needle insertion

Local skin infiltration and needle insertion may be undertaken at either the lateral or medial border of the transducer oriented transversly on the patient's thigh. Enough skin and subcutaneous infiltration should be utilized to minimize patient discomfort during needle manipulation.

A blunt-tipped block needle appropriate for the patient's size and tissue depth is advanced within the ultrasound beam's long axis (*in-plane* approach). The needle is introduced through the skin wheal passing

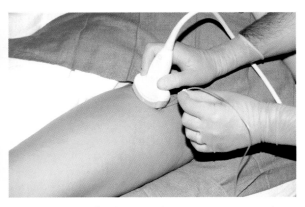

Figure 11.19 Needle placement during an anterior approach to sciatic nerve block.

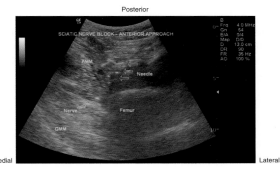

Figure 11.20 In-plane needle positioning during the placement of a sciatic nerve block via an anterior approach. AMM = adductor magnus muscle; GMM = gluteus maximus muscle.

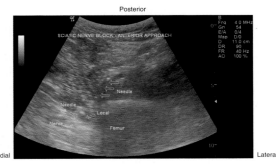

Figure 11.21 Local anesthetic injection during sciatic nerve block via an anterior approach. AMM = adductor magnus muscle.

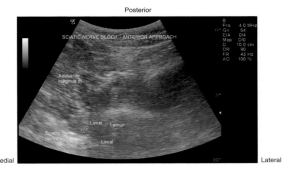

Figure 11.22 Local anesthetic in proximity to the sciatic nerve following nerve block via an anterior approach.

into the subcutaneous tissue and muscle while directed toward the sciatic nerve within the fascial plane between the hip adductor muscles and the gluteus maximus muscle (Figure 11.19). Look for the appearance of a hyperechoic line (needle) or tissue movement along the corresponding outer edge of the ultrasound screen as the needle is advanced (Figure 11.20).

Do not blindly advance the needle. If you are having difficulty identifying the needle's location, stop and look at your hands to make sure that you are passing straight through the beam of the ultrasound probe. If your needle appears to be in-plane with the beam, but remains hidden on the screen, you may need to make very small tilting or rotating movements with the probe to bring the needle into view. The initial image of your target structures should change very minimally, if at all. If the original scan has changed significantly in order to locate the needle, then remove the needle and begin again.

Local anesthetic injection and needle repositioning

The block needle should be placed in proximity to the nerve to pierce the surrounding fascia, without actually entering the nerve. The nerve itself will appear to be dissected away from the muscle as injection occurs ("hydrodissection"). During incremental injection, local anesthetic deposition should be visualized and monitored (Figure 11.21). A total of 20 to 40 ml of local anesthetic may be injected depending on the patient, as well as anesthetic type and concentration used. When finished, a pocket of anesthetic should be adjacent to, or, ideally, surrounding the nerve (Figure 11.22).

Additional considerations

When injection is undertaken, the needle tip does not have to be positioned on top of a nerve to block the nerve. In fact, doing so may risk injury. What is important is witnessing the *spread* of local anesthetic around the nerve requiring blockade, and this can sometimes be achieved with few needle reposition movements. The spread of the local anesthetic will appear as an expanding hypoechoic region in a well contained space.

A negative aspiration does not rule out an intravascular injection.

Remain alert to the possibility of intravascular injection if the spread of local anesthetic is not seen, as this may indicate that the local anesthetic is being deposited into a vessel.

Authors' clinical practice

- *Dosing regimen*: to maximize block duration for postoperative pain control while decreasing onset time for surgical anesthesia, we typically use 20 to 30 ml of 0.75% ropivacaine for proximal sciatic nerve blocks. The volume and dose of anesthetic used will be influenced by the patient, his/her history, relevant comorbid conditions, and the spread of local anesthetic.

- For cases in which extended postoperative analgesia will not be necessary, 1.5% or 2% mepivacaine with or without epinephrine is often substituted in 20 to 40 ml, depending on the patient and his/her history.

- Ultrasound-guided sciatic nerve blocks via the subgluteal or anterior approach can be technically challenging relative to other ultrasound-guided blocks as a result of the nerve's morphology at this level, the use of lower frequency probes, and the depth of tissue penetration required to complete the block. When first learning these approaches, use of a nerve stimulator can be helpful to confirm the nerve's position, especially in cases where the nerve is not imaged clearly.

- Careful consideration should be given to placement of proximal sciatic nerve blocks in patients who will require early recovery or function of their hamstring muscles. We do not routinely use these approaches in ambulatory foot/ankle cases in order to allow non-weight bearing patients to flex their knee while using crutches when they are discharged.

- Patients receiving any sciatic nerve block are at risk for falling after placement of the block. Consideration and discussion should take place with the patient prior to block placement, with instruction and follow-up provided postoperatively.

Suggested reading

Chan V W, Nova H, Abbas S, *et al.* (2006). Ultrasound examination and localization of the sciatic nerve: a volunteer study. *Anesthesiology*, **104**(2):309–14.

Sciatic nerve block: lateral popliteal fossa/distal thigh approach

Introduction and specific anatomy

The ultrasound-guided lateral popliteal fossa block of the sciatic nerve is a regional anesthetic approach for surgical procedures of the distal leg, foot, and ankle. This technique is performed at the most cephalad portion of the popliteal fossa or around the distal third of the thigh near the bifurcation of the sciatic nerve into its two common branches: the tibial and common peroneal nerves.

Sciatic nerve and branches

The sciatic nerve, the largest peripheral nerve in the human body, is formed from ventral roots of the lumbosacral plexus (L4–S3) (Figure 12.1). After exiting the pelvis via the greater sciatic foramen, the sciatic nerve travels in the posterior thigh deep to the long head of the biceps femoris muscle. Entering the popliteal space created by the hamstring and gastrocnemius muscles (semitendinosus muscle and semimembranosus muscle

Figure 12.1 Organization of the sacral plexus.

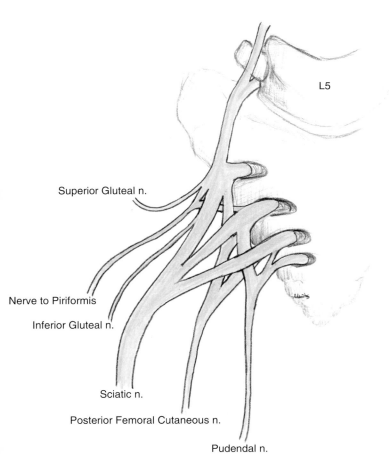

L5

Superior Gluteal n.

Nerve to Piriformis

Inferior Gluteal n.

Sciatic n.

Posterior Femoral Cutaneous n.

Pudendal n.

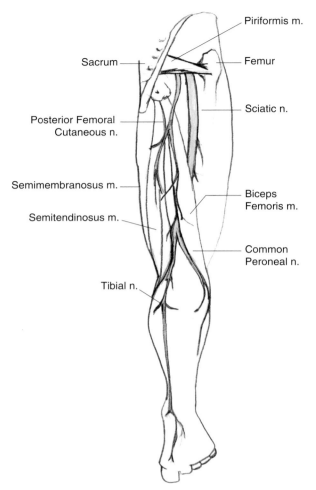

Figure 12.2 Posterior anatomy of the lower extremity with the sciatic nerve and its branches.

The *tibial nerve* (L4–S3), the larger of the two sciatic divisions, travels through the popliteal space lateral and posterior to the popliteal artery and vein before coursing medially into the lower leg behind the gastrocnemius muscle at the base of the fossa (Figure 12.2). The nerve follows a surface line down the leg from the center of the popliteal space to the midway point of the medial malleolus and the calcaneal tendon. The tibial nerve is responsible for muscular innervation of the calf (popliteus, gastrocnemius, and soleus muscles) and flexor muscles of the foot (tibialis posterior, flexor digitorum longus, and flexor hallicus longis muscles), provides articular branches to the knee, and branches that provide cutaneous innervation to most of the plantar portion of the foot and toes (Figure 12.5).

The *common peroneal nerve* (L4–S2) splits from the sciatic nerve and courses laterally across the popliteal space and around the fibular head and neck (Figure 12.2, Figure 12.4). The nerve travels distally behind the peroneus longus muscle along the lateral aspect of the lower leg only a short distance before dividing into the deep and superficial peroneal nerves.

The *deep peroneal nerve* descends deep to the muscles of the anterior leg along the interosseous membrane between the tibia and fibula. In the lower third of the leg, the deep peroneal nerve joins with the anterior tibial artery, crossing the ankle joint deep to the extensor retinaculum. The nerve is adjacent to the vessels at the ankle (Figure 12.4). The deep peroneal nerve provides motor innervation to extensor muscles of the foot and ankle along with sensory innervation to the ankle joint and the web space between the first and second toes.

The *superficial peroneal nerve* travels deep to the peroneal muscles, becoming superficial at about the mid-portion of the lower leg (Figure 12.4). The nerve provides motor innervation to muscles of the lateral leg and ankle (peroneus longus and brevis muscles) and sensory innervation to the lateral leg and dorsum of the foot.

The *sural nerve* also provides cutaneous innervation to inferior portions of the lateral and posterior lower leg as well as the lateral aspect of the foot (Figure 12.5). The nerve typically forms along the lateral leg from cutaneous branches of both the tibial and common peroneal nerves (See also Chapter 10: Lower extremity anatomy for regional anesthesia). The sural nerve travels distally within deep fascia prior to becoming superficial and coursing around the posterior portion of the lateral malleolus.

superomedially; biceps femoris long head muscle superolaterally; medial and lateral heads of the gastrocnemius muscle inferiorly), the sciatic nerve divides to form the tibial nerve medially, and the common peroneal nerve laterally. The point where this bifurcation occurs is variable but generally occurs around the distal 2/3 portion of the patient's thigh, proximal to the popliteal space (Figures 12.2 and 12.3).

The main terminal branches of the sciatic nerve providing motor and sensory innervation to the leg, ankle, and foot include the superficial and deep peroneal nerves (from the common peroneal nerve), the posterior tibial nerve (ending as calcaneal and plantar nerves of the foot), and the sural nerve (see also Chapter 10: Lower extremity anatomy for regional anesthesia).

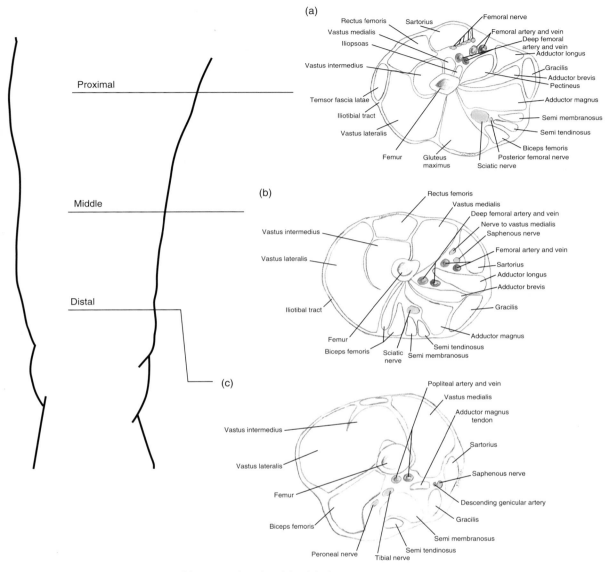

Figure 12.3 Cross-sectional anatomy of the proximal, mid, and distal thigh.

The saphenous nerve

The saphenous nerve is a distal continuation of the femoral nerve that provides cutaneous innervation to medial portions of the leg, ankle, and foot (Figure 12.5). It is the only branch of the femoral nerve that must be accounted for below the knee.

The saphenous nerve originates proximally in the thigh descending through the femoral triangle lateral to the femoral vessels. The nerve courses distally with the femoral artery in the adductor canal deep to the sartorius muscle before emerging in the distal thigh between the sartorius and gracilis muscles. The nerve then becomes superficial as it passes into the leg over the medial border of the knee. From here the nerve consistently travels with the great saphenous vein toward the medial ankle, sending cutaneous branches to the anteromedial and posteromedial leg along the way.

103

Proper blockade of the sciatic nerve along with the saphenous nerve will provide complete anesthesia of the foot and ankle.

Ultrasound anatomy

Orienting structure: popliteal artery and biceps femoris muscle

An appreciation of the muscles, vessels, and fascial planes within the distal thigh and popliteal space will facilitate ultrasound imaging and target location with this block (Figure 12.6). The orienting structures for this block are the popliteal artery (near the popliteal space) and the biceps femoris muscle.

Placing the transducer transversly across the apex of the popliteal space (see also Technique description/ Scanning), the popliteal artery and vein may be visualized close to the femur. The sciatic nerve (or its individual trunks) will be lateral and posterior to the vessels (Figure 12.6).

Moving the probe to a more proximal position around the 2/3 distal portion of the thigh (Figure 12.7a and b), the sciatic nerve typically appears as an anisotropic round *ball*. This differs from more proximal ultrasound approaches to the sciatic nerve where the nerve may actually have a flattened appearance. The nerve is situated along the anterior (deep to) or medial border of the biceps femoris muscle within the fascial plane separating the hamstring muscles (Figure 12.8).

Table 12.1 shows some sample operative procedures for consideration of ultrasound-guided lateral popliteal sciatic nerve block.

Contraindications

Table 12.2 lists contraindications to ultrasound-guided lateral popliteal sciatic nerve block.

Side effects and complications

Table 12.3 shows some side effects and complications associated with ultrasound-guided lateral popliteal sciatic nerve block.

Equipment

- Ultrasound machine with *high-frequency* (10 to 12 MHz) *linear array* probe
- Sterile skin preparation (e.g., betadine, chlorhexidine)

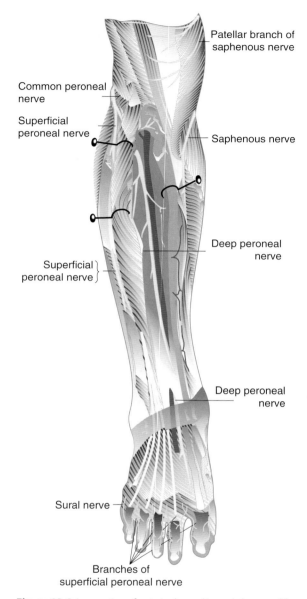

Figure 12.4 Innervation of anterior leg, ankle, and dorsum of foot.

- 10-cm, blunt-tipped needle (large or obese patients may require a 15-cm needle)
- Sterile cover for ultrasound probe
- Sterile ultrasound gel
- Local anesthetic for a skin wheal and subcutaneous infiltration
- Sterile gloves
- Appropriate local anesthetic and volume in 20-ml syringes

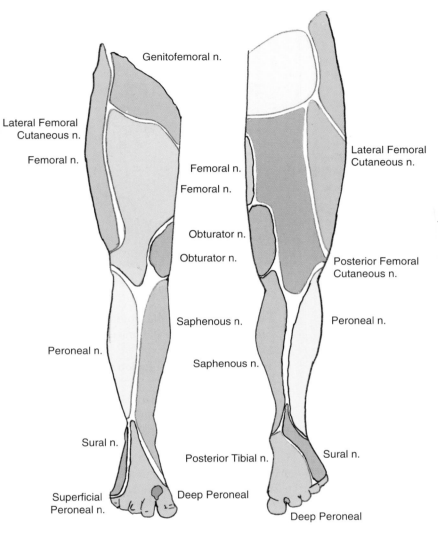

Figure 12.5 Sensory nerve distribution to the lower extremity.

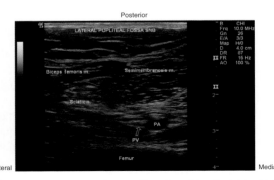

Figure 12.6 Transverse ultrasound imaging of the distal right thigh near the popliteal apex with the popliteal artery and vein (collapsed) identified. PA = popliteal artery; PV = popliteal vein.

Structures that are required to be identified	Structures that may be seen
Sciatic nerve (tibial nerve/ common peroneal nerve) Popliteal artery	Semimembranosis muscle Semitendonosis muscle
Biceps femoris muscle Separation of the sciatic nerve into tibial and common peroneal nerves	Popliteal vein Femur Fascia

105

(a)

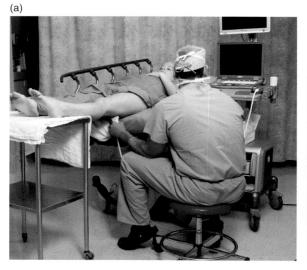

(b)

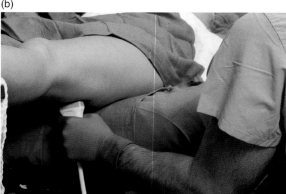

Figures 12.7 (a) and (b) Transducer positioned under the distal thigh for left lateral popliteal sciatic nerve block (gapped-supine positioning).

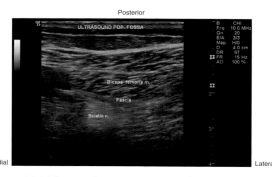

Figure 12.8 Ultrasound transverse imaging of the distal left thigh above the popliteal space prior to the separation of the common peroneal and tibial nerves.

Pillows or a reusable block platform for leg elevation *or* a block table with appropriate padding for leg support during gapped-supine positioning

- Appropriate sedation, monitoring, and oxygen supply
- Illustrated in Figure 12.9

Technique

Technique summary

1. Monitors placed and patient appropriately sedated
2. Sterile preparation applied to procedural site
3. Clear, sterile adhesive cover applied to ultrasound probe

4. Perform systematic ultrasound scan to find optimal location for placement of nerve block
5. Skin wheal is raised
6. Insert block needle and guide toward target structures
7. Inject local anesthetic
8. Reposition needle as necessary to complete block

Scanning

The lateral popliteal/distal thigh sciatic nerve block may be performed in a number of different patient positions including prone, lateral, semi-lateral and supine. We routinely use and teach the single-shot lateral popliteal sciatic nerve block with the patient in the supine position.

The ultrasound machine is placed at the head of the bed next to the patient on the same side to be blocked. With the physician facing the machine, the hand closest to the patient manipulates the ultrasound probe.

Thus for a *left* sciatic lateral popliteal block, the operator performs the ultrasound scan with their left hand while guiding the block needle with the right hand (Figure 12.16).

The patient's popliteal fossa and distal thigh are exposed by using one of two positioning techniques for the supine patient. *Gapped-supine* positioning involves moving the patient near the end of the bed with both knees kept in a neutral position while resting the patient's legs on a stable platform or table. This essentially creates an exposed "gap" beneath the

Table 12.1 Sample operative procedures for consideration of ultrasound-guided lateral popliteal sciatic nerve block

Procedure		Supplemental block[1]
Procedures involving multiple toes, midfoot, or forefoot	R	Saphenous nerve for procedures of medial midfoot or forefoot
Procedures involving calcaneus or calcaneal (Achilles) tendon	R	Saphenous nerve
Procedures of the ankle	R	Saphenous nerve
Procedures of the distal leg	R	Saphenous nerve
Procedures of the mid leg[2]	M	Saphenous nerve
Procedures of proximal leg	NR	–

Notes: R = recommended; M = maybe; NR = not recommended
[1]Consideration should be made for tourniquet position and use.
[2]Block placement may need to be shifted proximally on the thigh (e.g., midfemoral or other approach) from where routine lateral popliteal fossa block is placed.

Table 12.2 Contraindications to ultrasound-guided lateral popliteal sciatic nerve block

Absolute contraindications	Relative contraindications
Patient refusal	Ipsilateral neuromuscular disease/damage
Infection over site of needle insertion	Contralateral neuromuscular disease/damage in ambulatory patient
Allergy to local anesthetics	Anticoagulation or bleeding disorder

Table 12.3 Side effects and complications associated with ultrasound-guided lateral popliteal sciatic nerve block

Side effects	Complications[1]
Motor blockade of foot and ankle for partial duration of local anesthetic effect	
Patient is at fall risk following block placement until block resolution	

Note: [1]Infection, nerve damage, local anesthetic toxicity, vascular injury, or hematoma are potential complications common to all nerve blocks.

patient's calf to mid-thigh (Figure 12.10). A draw sheet should be kept under the patient in order to facilitate positioning by two persons.

The gapped-supine positioning technique provides a flat, open surface for the transducer probe to be manipulated. Additionally, the patient is kept supine to allow easy access to the airway should it be necessary. Gapped-supine positioning is limited mainly by the time and manpower constraints of repositioning the patient in the bed before and after the block. An adequate amount of room is also necessary to have the patient positioned at the end of the bed safely and discretely if other patients are nearby.

Alternatively, the *leg elevation technique* exposes the popliteal space and distal thigh by elevating the leg to be blocked onto pillows or a few blankets. Slight flexion of the knee should be allowed, creating just enough room for the ultrasound probe to be placed and manipulated beneath the patient's thigh (Figure 12.11).

The leg-elevation technique avoids excessive repositioning time, is generally not uncomfortable for the patient, and can easily be done by the sole practitioner. In addition, the head of the bed can be slightly elevated if necessary while the airway is left easily accessible. The leg elevation technique may be limited by the tendency for the limb to "roll" or externally rotate without support while raised on pillows. Ultrasound imaging and probe manipulation may also be technically more difficult in the restricted space (or on the angled surface) between the patient's thigh and the bed, especially in obese patients.

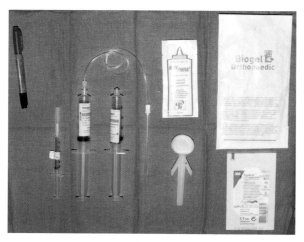

Figure 12.9 Equipment tray prepared for ultrasound-guided sciatic nerve block.

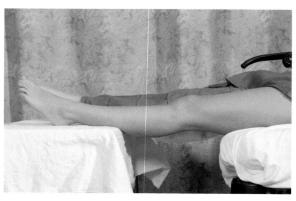

Figure 12.10 Gapped-supine positioning for lateral popliteal sciatic nerve block.

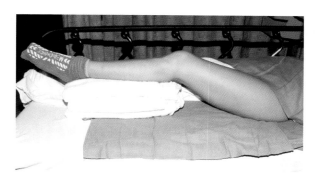

Figure 12.11 Leg-elevation positioning for lateral popliteal sciatic nerve block.

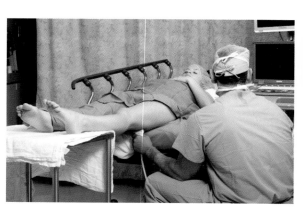

Figure 12.12 Scanning using gapped-supine positioning.

Additional considerations

When positioning using the leg-elevation technique, take care not to flex the knee too much as it is raised.

Only enough room between the patient's posterior thigh and the bed should be created for probe insertion and subtle manipulation. In fact, the weight of the patient's leg resting on the upright probe can often be helpful as additional upward pressure on the probe becomes less necessary.

Prior to beginning the scan, the lateral portion of the patient's distal thigh is disinfected with a sterile preparation solution. We routinely place a protective covering over the ultrasound transducer to minimize patient-to-patient contact, although the probe is not in the immediate proximity of the sterile needle with this approach.

The ultrasound probe is placed transversely under the posterior aspect of the patient's distal thigh at the proximal apex of the popliteal space to create a transverse image of the structures crossing the ultrasound beam (Figures 12.12 and 12.13). By convention, the probe should be oriented such that the probe indicator is directed to the patient's right.

Additional considerations

The sciatic nerve or separate tibial and common peroneal nerves may be imaged to complete a single-shot block. The image obtained is dependent on the patient's relative anatomy and how far distally along the thigh the transducer is positioned (Figure 12.14a, b and c).

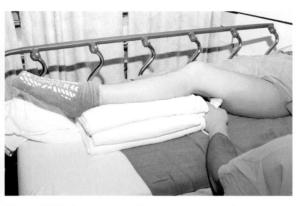

Figure 12.13 Scanning using leg-elevation positioning.

"Following the nerve" up and down the distal thigh a short distance can be helpful to identify the nerve's position and confirm the best position for needle placement.

It may be important to ensure that an identified single nerve structure is not simply the tibial nerve with the common peroneal component having branched higher in the thigh. This misidentification may be a possible reason for only partial set up of the block.

Scanning should be performed in a systematic manner (i.e., systematic scan) with steady, anteriorly directed pressure placed on the probe. Start by placing the probe beneath the patient's thigh in the popliteal fossa or apex and making small medial adjustments until the probe is centered under the leg. Note the anatomy imaged on the ultrasound screen as the probe is moved.

Attempt to identify the popliteal artery at the starting position near the popliteal apex. The nerve is typically found lateral and posterior relative to the artery (Figure 12.6), and may appear as separate tibial and common peroneal nerve components at this distal location.

Begin to slowly scan away from the popliteal space proximally, keeping the nerve(s) in view and identify the biceps femoris muscle. The muscle belly is anatomically lateral and posterior to the sciatic nerve (Figure 12.15). The branching location of the common peroneal and tibial nerves may also be identified depending on the patient's anatomy.

At the mid-distal thigh position, the sciatic nerve typically lies within a fascial plane that

(a)
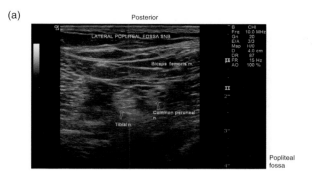

(b)
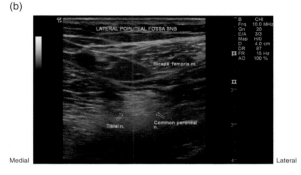

(c)
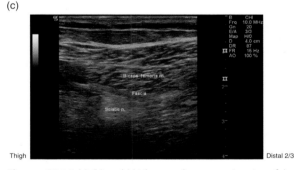

Figures 12.14 (a), (b), and (c) Ultrasound transverse imaging of the left thigh moving proximally from the popliteal apex to identify the convergence of tibial and common peroneal nerves.

separates the hamstring muscles and appears as a round ball structure. Keep in mind, the nerve will characteristically exhibit anisotropy: the neural and connective tissue will vary in echogenicity consistent with changes in the angle of incidence at which the nerve is imaged (See Chapter 2: Introduction to ultrasound). Thus, subtle tilting or rotating changes in the angle of the probe may alter the appearance of the nerve on the screen, making it more or less visible.

109

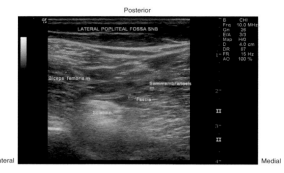

Figure 12.15 Ultrasound transverse imaging of the distal right thigh above the popliteal space prior to separation of the common peroneal and tibial nerves.

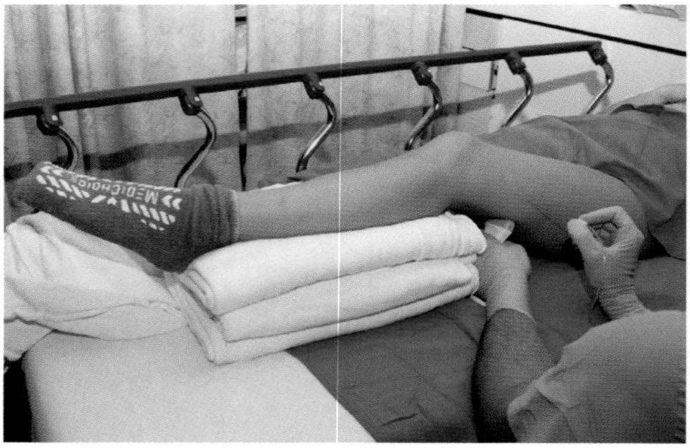

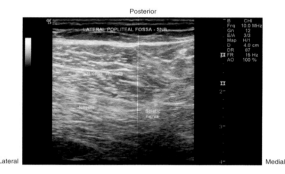

Figure 12.16 In-plane needle insertion (leg-elevation positioning).

Additional considerations

To optimize the quality of the transverse image, subtle manipulations of the transducer are often necessary. These manipulations may involve small changes in probe-tip direction (tilting, rotating, or sliding) and/or varying pressure applied to the probe during scanning.

Varying the amount of pressure applied to the probe can be a useful tool in helping to identify the sciatic nerve. The nerve is less compressible than the surrounding muscle and fat, and with varied pressure on the transducer, one can often see the nerve move up and down as this pressure is applied and relaxed.

Figure 12.17 Block needle approaching the sciatic nerve during block of the right lower extremity via a lateral popliteal approach.

Once an ideal location for block placement is found, it is important to maintain the probe's position. When the patient is in the gapped-supine position, the arm the physician uses to perform the scan should be comfortably stabilized by resting the elbow on the ipsilateral knee under the patient's leg (Figure 12.12). Using the leg-elevation technique, the probe is stabilized by the bed and the weight of the patient's leg, with the operator's fist around the distal end of the probe to protect the connection point between the cord and the transducer (Figure 12.13).

Needle insertion

Having identified the sciatic nerve at the appropriate level, skin and subcutaneous infiltration is undertaken on the lateral thigh relative to the position of the ultrasound probe.

A blunt tipped block needle is then directed in-plane with the ultrasound beam (Figures 12.16 and 12.17). The initial direction of needle advancement should be parallel to the ultrasound probe in order to facilitate identification of the needle's direction and depth. Look for the appearance of a hyperechoic line (needle) or tissue movement along the lateral edge of the ultrasound screen as the needle is advanced.

Do not blindly advance the needle. If you are having difficulty identifying the needle's location, stop and look at your hands to make sure that you are passing straight through the beam of the ultrasound probe. If your needle appears to be in plane with the beam, but remains hidden on the screen, you may need to make very small tilting or rotating movements with the probe to bring the needle into view. The initial image of your target structures should change very minimally, if at all. If the original scan has changed significantly in order to locate the needle, then remove the needle and begin again.

(a) 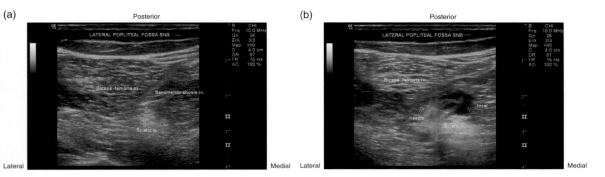 (b)

Figures 12.18 (a) and (b) Local anesthetic injection with "hydrodissection" of the nerve away from fascia and muscle during a lateral popliteal block approach to the sciatic nerve.

Additional considerations

When difficulty in identifying the needle tip continues to be encountered, a *small* amount of local anesthetic (1 or 2 ml) may also be injected while monitoring for tissue changes ("hydrolocation"). By changing the echogenicity of the surrounding tissue, hydrolocation may make needle-tip identification easier in some cases. If the injection is not observed on the ultrasound screen, however, it should be immediately stopped.

Though hydrolocation may be helpful at times, we do not advocate its routine use as a substitute for proper hand and needle positioning technique when performing an in-plane approach.

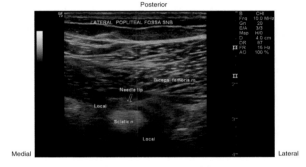

Figure 12.19 Completing injection around the sciatic nerve during a lateral popliteal approach of the left lower extremity (e.g., "donut sign").

Once oriented, the needle tip can be redirected in an anterior or posterior direction as necessary to approach the sciatic nerve.

Local anesthetic injection and needle repositioning

The block needle should be placed in proximity to the nerve to pierce the surrounding fascia, without actually entering the nerve. The nerve will appear to be dissected away from the muscle by the expanding, hypoechoic pocket of anesthetic as injection occurs ("hydrodissection") (Figure 12.18a and b). Perform the injection in 3- to 5-ml increments with aspirations attempted between injections to ensure the needle tip remains extravascular. Remember, anesthetic spread should *always* be observed under ultrasound. Failure to visualize the anesthetic during injection should prompt the operator to stop

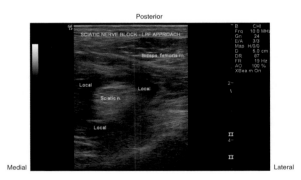

Figure 12.20 Local anesthetic surrounding the sciatic nerve during a lateral popliteal approach of the left lower extremity.

injecting immediately, regardless of a prior negative aspiration.

Ideally, the nerve should be completely surrounded with anesthetic when finished (e.g., "donut sign" or "eyeball sign") (Figures 12.19 and 12.20).

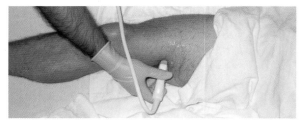

Figure 12.21 Patient and probe positioning for perifemoral transsartorial saphenous nerve block.

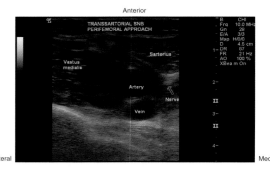

Figure 12.22 Ultrasound imaging of mid-distal thigh for perifemoral transsartorial saphenous nerve block.

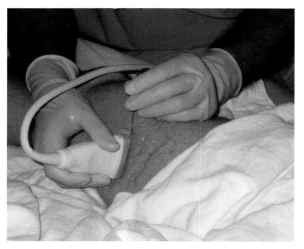

Figure 12.23 In-plane needle insertion for perifemoral transsartorial saphenous nerve block.

Saphenous nerve blocks

For procedures involving the medial foot, ankle, or distal leg, blockade of the saphenous nerve will be necessary to provide proper anesthesia and/or analgesia when performing a regional technique. The saphenous nerve can be approached for ultrasound-guided blockade at multiple points from its origin in the proximal thigh down to the medial ankle.

Because the nerve is small, it may be difficult to visualize with ultrasound depending on the patient and physician experience level. Thus, these approaches described may at times rely more on placement of anesthetic in a proper tissue plane rather than imaging the nerve directly.

Transsartorial (perifemoral) approach

This block is performed along the medial aspect of the mid-distal thigh where the saphenous nerve travels in the adductor canal with the femoral artery prior to the artery leaving the canal via the adductor hiatus. *The orienting structure for this block is the femoral artery.*

The patient is kept supine with a small amount of external rotation at the hip on the side to be blocked. The anteromedial distal thigh is cleaned with a sterile preparation solution. Scanning is undertaken by placing a high-frequency probe transversly along the anteromedial thigh, approximately 8 to 10 cm proximal to the patella. Look for the hyperechoic edge of the femur, then scan medially with small adjustments to identify the femoral artery at this initial location (Figure 12.21). Pulse-wave Doppler or color-flow imaging can be helpful in identifying the artery's position.

Keeping the femoral artery in view, scan distally to identify the point at which the femoral artery leaves the adductor canal, becoming the popliteal artery. The artery will begin to course posteriorly at this point, to the bottom of the image. Where this transition begins to occur is typically the location for block placement (Figure 12.22).

The saphenous nerve may travel with other small nerves at this location (e.g., the nerve to the vastus medialis), and therefore the nerve structure may be large enough to be visualized at this location just medial or superficial to the artery.

A small skin wheal is placed at the lateral (anterior) border of the transducer, and a blunt bevel block needle is introduced in plane toward the medial aspect of the femoral artery (Figure 12.23). An out-of-plane technique may also be used.

Local anesthetic is injected deep to the sartorius muscle and medial to the femoral artery to complete the block. Five to 10 ml of local anesthetic is usually required (Figure 12.24).

The benefits of the transsartorial perifemoral approach include the presence of a highly visible orienting structure (femoral artery), increased potential to visualize the target nerve, and reliable blockade when placed appropriately.

One potential limitation, however, is possible motor involvement of the vastus medialis muscle. This should be carefully considered, and the effects (the potential for some quadriceps weakness) discussed with the patient, prior to placement.

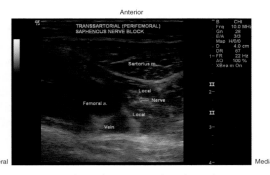

Figure 12.24 Local anesthetic surrounding the saphenous nerve, perifemoral transsartorial saphenous nerve block.

Transsartorial (distal thigh) approach

The saphenous nerve may also be blocked just above the knee as the nerve travels within the fascial plane separating the sartorius and vastus medialis muscles. The block is slightly different from the transsartorial perifemoral approach in that a major vascular landmark is often lacking, and the nerve usually tends to be less visible at this level. By separating the sartorius and vastus medialis muscle planes with local anesthetic, blockade of the saphenous nerve can be achieved with reasonable success.

With the patient positioned supine, a high-frequency tranducer is placed just above the patella to image the femur. The probe is then slowly moved to the medial side of the leg above the medial epicondyle of the femur while noting the muscle changes on the ultrasound screen (Figure 12.25a). The vastus medialis muscle will be first to appear. As the probe continues to be moved medially, the sartorius muscle should come into view. The muscular separation between the sartorius muscle and vastus medialis muscle is the location for anesthetic injection (Figure 12.26). At times, the descending genicular artery may be visualized close to the nerve.

For this block, we often choose an out-of-plane needle approach to insert the needle more directly

(a)

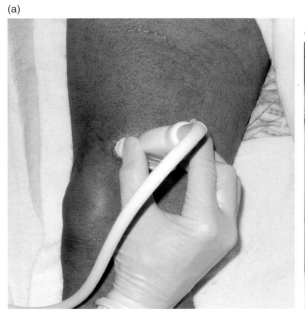

(b)

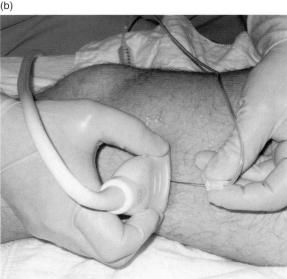

Figure 12.25 (a) and (b) Probe positioning and out-of-plane needle insertion for distal thigh transsartorial saphenous nerve block.

into the fascial plane without traversing the muscle bellies (Figure 12.25b).

Perivenous approach

The saphenous nerve may also be reliably blocked with ultrasound guidance at a point just below the knee and medial to the tibial tuberosity.

At this level, the saphenous nerve consistently travels with the saphenous vein, though its position around the vein may be variable. Therefore, for this approach, *the orienting structure is the saphenous vein.* The goal is to place anesthetic *around* the saphenous *vein,* as the saphenous nerve will not always be easily visualized.

A light tourniquet is placed around the distal thigh in order to facilitate dilation of the vein distally if necessary. At the level of the tibial tuberosity, the antero-medial leg is disinfected with antiseptic solution, and a high-frequency transducer, prepared with a sterile cover, and conduction gel, is used to identify the saphenous vein. The probe should be oriented to obtain a transverse image of the vessel as it crosses the ultrasound beam (Figure 12.27a and b).

The vein will be very superficial at this level, typically not more than a centimeter deep, and easily collapsed if excessive pressure is placed on the ultrasound probe. The vein should be followed distally with ultrasound along the medial border of the leg to confirm its identity and position. This may be particulary important in individuals where the vein is not readily apparent from visual inspection of their surface anatomy.

A control syringe with a 25-gauge needle, or a syringe with a blunt bevel block needle may be used to complete the block. The needle is passed under the transducer at the lateral side of the patient's leg, toward the saphenous vein. Due to the superficial nature of the vein, and the lack of muscle tissue at this location, the block needle should be easily visualized as it is passed (Figure 12.28). Care must be taken to avoid puncturing the vein while local anesthetic is deposited around the vessel. The vein should be completely surrounded with anesthetic when finished. Typically 5 to 10 ml of local anesthetic is necessary (Figure 12.29).

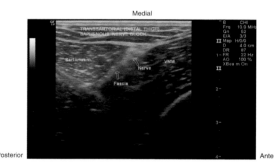

Figure 12.26 Site (fascia) for local anesthetic injection, transsartorial (distal thigh) approach. VVM = vastus medialis muscle.

Field block at the ankle

For procedures of the foot, the nerve can be easily blocked with a subcutaneous injection of 5 to 10 ml of local anesthetic across the medial leg just above the medial malleolus (Figure 12.30). Due to the multiple subcutaneous branches of the saphenous nerve, this may be the preferable way to approach this block for cases of the medial foot without involvement of the ankle or distal leg.

(a)

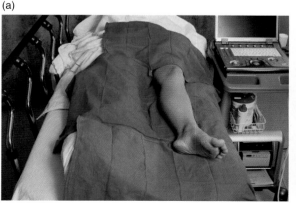

(b)

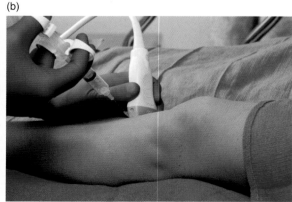

Figure 12.27 (a) and (b) Positioning and placement of perivenous saphenous nerve block in the proximal portion of the leg.

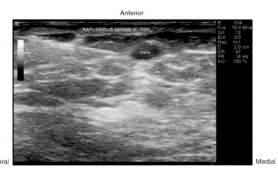

Figure 12.28 Blocking the saphenous nerve at the level of the tibial tuberosity (perivenous approach).

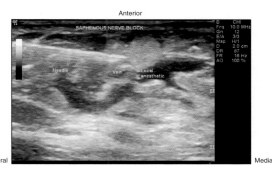

Figure 12.29 Completing injection of local anesthetic around the saphenous vein during saphenous nerve block at the level of tibial tuberosity (perivenous approach).

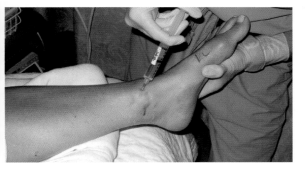

Figure 12.30 Saphenous nerve field block at the ankle.

Authors' clinical practice

- Dosing regimen: to maximize block duration for postoperative pain control while decreasing onset time for surgical anesthesia, we typically use 30 to 40 ml of 0.75% ropivacaine for our lateral popliteal fossa/distal thigh sciatic nerve blocks. The volume and dose of anesthetic used will be influenced by the patient, his/her history, relevant comorbid conditions, and the spread of local anesthetic.

- For cases in which extended postoperative analgesia will not be necessary, mepivacaine with or without epinephrine is often substituted in 20- to 40-ml volumes.

- We prefer to keep patients supine for placement of *single-shot* distal sciatic nerve blocks to allow for improved patient comfort and the relative convenience of an easily accessible airway. For distal (and proximal) sciatic perineural catheters, we find the lateral decubitus position allows for a larger ultrasound scanning area along the posterior thigh and a more manageable

surface for catheter insertion by the sole practioner (See Chapter 19: Sciatic continuous perineural catheters).

- Consideration should be given to the surgeon's use of a pneumatic tourniquet when considering a regional anesthetic of the leg. The use and/or location of the tourniquet (ankle vs. calf vs. thigh) will determine the need for supplementary nerve blocks and additional sedation requirements during the surgical case.

- Patients receiving any sciatic nerve block are at risk for falling after placement of the block. Discussion and consideration should take place with the patient prior to block placement, with instruction and follow-up provided postoperatively.

Suggested reading

Dayan V, Cura L, Cubas S, Carriquiry G. (2008). Surgical anatomy of the saphenous nerve. *Ann Thorac Surg*, 85(3):896–900.

Khabiri B, Arbona F, Norton J. (2007). "Gapped supine" position for ultrasound guided lateral popliteal fossa block of the sciatic nerve. *Anesth Analg*, 105(5):1519.

Krombach J, Gray A T. (2009). Reply to Drs. Tsui and Ozelsel. *Reg Anesth Pain Med*, 34(2):178.

Sinha A, Chan V W. (2004). Ultrasound imaging for popliteal sciatic nerve block. *Reg Anesth Pain Med*, 29(2):130–4.

Tsui B C, Finucane B T. (2006). The importance of ultrasound landmarks: a "traceback" approach using the popliteal blood vessels for identification of the sciatic nerve. *Reg Anesth Pain Med*, 31(5):481–2.

Tsui B C, Ozelsel T. (2009). Ultrasound-guided transsartorial perifemoral artery approach for saphenous nerve block. *Reg Anesth Pain Med*, 34(2):177–8.

Chapter 13

Femoral peripheral nerve block

Introduction and specific anatomy

Femoral nerve

The ultrasound-guided femoral nerve block is a relatively simple block to perform, but useful in multiple clinical settings. It can be used to supply anesthesia to the anterior thigh and knee, or to supply analgesia for femur and knee surgery, as well as hip procedures, especially when larger volumes are injected, as in a "3-in-1 block". The femoral nerve originates as the largest branch off the lumbar plexus, and comprises branches from the second, third, and fourth lumbar nerves (Figure 13.1). It passes through the psoas muscle, then travels down toward the leg within the groove formed between the psoas and ilacus muscles. The nerve then passes down into the anterior portion of the thigh under the inguinal ligament, and travels immediately lateral to the femoral artery (Figures 13.2 and 13.3). Near the level of the femoral crease, the femoral nerve is covered by the fascia lata and fascia iliaca and separated from the femoral artery and vein by the iliopectineal ligament (Figure 13.4). This physical separation of the femoral nerve from the vascular structures allows for a more contained injection of local anesthetic when performing the nerve block. As the femoral nerve travels distally past the inguinal ligament and crease, it separates into a more superficial anterior division, which is primarily sensory, and a deeper posterior division, which is primarily motor (Table 13.1). The sensory branches of the femoral nerve innervate the anterior and medial thigh, the medial leg down to the ankle, and provide articular innervation to the hip and knee (Figure 13.5). The motor branches innervate the individual heads of the quadriceps muscles, the sartorius muscle, and supply branches to the ilacus and pectineus muscles.

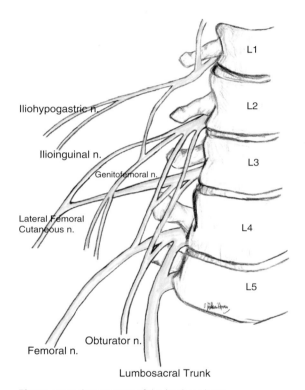

Figure 13.1 Organization of the lumbar plexus.

"3-in-1" block

This block was initially described by Winnie *et al.* (1973) as a low approach to a lumbar plexus block by essentially increasing the total volume injected during a femoral nerve block. The authors hypothesized that the increased local anesthetic volume would travel proximally within the fascial layer to anesthetize the femoral, obturator, and lateral femoral cutaneous nerves. This theory has not been confirmed clinically or radiographically, but this approach remains in high use clinically. The "3-in-1" nerve block seldom does as

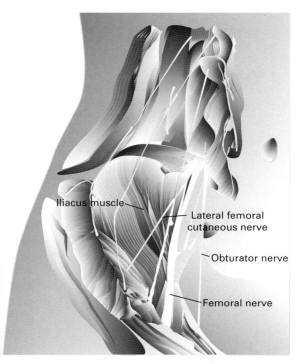

Figure 13.2 Dissection of the lumbar plexus, with the psoas muscle removed.

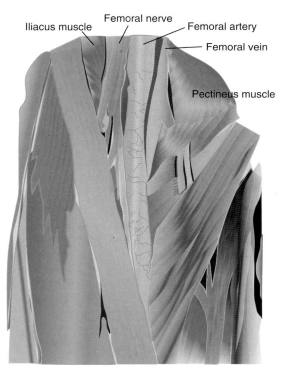

Figure 13.3 Dissection of the femoral triangle.

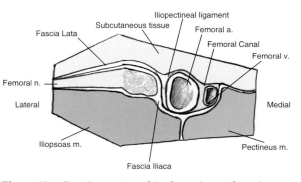

Figure 13.4 Fascial separation of the femoral nerve from the femoral artery and vein.

Table 13.1 Innervation of anterior and posterior divisions of the femoral nerve

Anterior division	*Sensory*: anterior femoral cutaneous nerves (anterior thigh)
	Motor: branch to sartorius muscle
Posterior division	*Sensory*: saphenous nerve (medial leg)
	Motor: branches to individual muscles of the quadriceps
	Articular: branches to anterior hip and majority of knee

its name implies. Nerve stimulator data show that it produces a reliable femoral nerve block (~90%), an occasional block of the lateral femoral cutaneous nerve (~60 to 70%), and an unreliable obturator nerve block (<50%). This may be because, as proposed, the local anesthetic spreads laterally under the ilacus fascia to the lateral femoral cutaneous nerve, but it does not have significant spread cephalad or medially to reach the obturator nerve consistently. Therefore, this block has been considered more along the lines of the "2-in-1" or "2½-in-1" block, rather than a "3-in-1" block.

Femoral vasculature

The femoral artery and vein travel parallel to the femoral nerve, and are located medially to the nerve. The mnemonic NAVEL (nerve, artery, vein, empty space, and lymphatics) is useful when

117

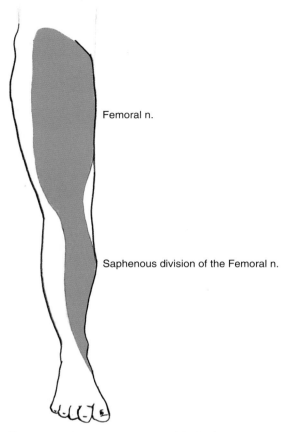

Femoral n.

Saphenous division of the Femoral n.

Figure 13.5 Cutaneous innervation of the lumbar plexus.

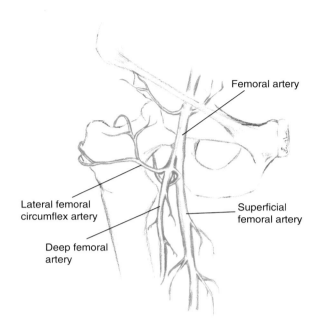

Femoral artery

Lateral femoral
circumflex artery

Superficial
femoral artery

Deep femoral
artery

Figure 13.6 Branching of the profunda femoris and lateral circumflex femoral arteries.

from the femoral artery, proximal to the take-off from the profunda femoris, bringing it closer to the level of the inguinal crease.

Additional considerations

The lateral femoral circumflex artery has been found to have origination from the femoral artery as frequently as 22.7% of the time.

Some investigations have found that the lateral femoral circumflex artery occurred within 1 cm of the inguinal crease 50% of the time.

There is no difference between sexes or sides when the lateral circumflex femoral artery originates from the femoral artery.

---

remembering the lateral to medial relationship of these structures.

Near the level of the inguinal crease, typically within 1 to 2 cm, the femoral artery branches as the profunda femoris artery, and continues as the superficial femoral artery (Figure 13.6). The superficial femoral artery continues to travel medial to the nerve within the femoral triangle. The profunda femoris artery initially travels just posterior, or deep, to the femoral nerve before diving deeper. Just as the profunda femoris artery emerges from the femoral artery, it usually gives off a branch as the lateral circumflex femoral artery (Figure 13.6). A high incidence of variation in this artery's origination occurs, though. It is not uncommon for the lateral circumflex femoral artery to have a direct take-off from the femoral artery, either above or below the origin of the profunda femoris artery. Ten percent to 20% of the time, the lateral circumflex femoral artery arises directly

Ultrasound anatomy

Orienting structure: femoral artery (Figure 13.7)

The orienting structure to perform this block is the *femoral artery* (Figure 13.8). At the site where the scanning and procedure are performed, the ultrasound image will show the femoral nerve located immediately lateral to the femoral artery, and just medial to the iliopsoas muscle. The femoral vein is located medial to the femoral artery.

Anterior

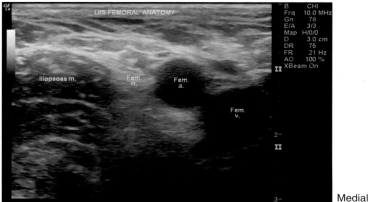

Lateral

Posterior

Medial

Figure 13.7 Normal femoral ultrasound anatomy near the inguinal crease.

Structures that are required to be identified	Structures that may be seen
Femoral artery	Iliopsoas muscle
Femoral vein	Profunda femoris artery
Femoral nerve	Lateral femoral circumflex artery
	Anomalous vasculature

Additional considerations

If more than one artery is seen on the initial scan, it may be either the profunda femoris or the lateral circumflex femoral artery in view. Scanning more *proximal* in the inguinal region can result in a position at a site before these arteries branch off the femoral artery.

Table 13.2 shows some sample operative procedures for consideration of a femoral or "3-in-1" nerve block.

Contraindications

Table 13.3 shows some contraindications to a femoral nerve block.

Side effects and complications

Table 13.4 shows some side effects and complications associated with a femoral nerve block.

Equipment

- Ultrasound machine
- High-frequency linear array ultrasound probe

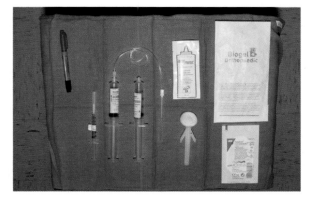

Figure 13.8 Equipment required for the performance of ultrasound-guided femoral nerve block.

- Sterile skin preparation
- 4- to 5-cm, blunt-tipped needle (may need a longer needle for very obese patients)
- Ultrasound probe cover
- Sterile ultrasound gel
- Local anesthetic for skin infiltration at block needle insertion site
- Sterile gloves
- Appropriate local anesthetic and volume in 20-ml syringes
- Illustrated in Figure 13.9

Technique
Scanning

The patient should be positioned supine with his/her arms resting comfortably across his/her chest or

119

Table 13.2 Sample operative procedures for consideration of femoral or "3-in-1" nerve block

Procedure		Supplemental block
Total hip arthropathy	R	+/− Obturator nerve, +/− Lateral femoral cutaneous nerve
Hip arthroscopy	R	+/− Obturator nerve
Femur procedures	R	−
Quadriceps procedures (e.g., biopsy, tendon repair)	R	−
Total knee arthropathy	R	+/− Sciatic nerve
Ligament surgery of the knee, including anterior cruciate ligament (ACL) reconstruction[1]	R	+/− Sciatic nerve[1]
Knee arthroscopy	R	−
Open meniscal repairs	R	−
Saphenous vein stripping, including below the knee	M	−
Tibial procedures	NR	−
Procedures of the foot and ankle	NR	−

Note: R = recommended; M = maybe; NR = not recommended
[1]When the ACL is an allograft from the hamstring tendon, the tendon harvest falls in the sciatic nerve distribution.

Table 13.3 Contraindications to femoral nerve block

Absolute contraindications	Relative contraindications
Patient refusal	Ipsilateral neuromuscular disease/damage
Infection over site of needle insertion	Anticoagulation or bleeding disorder[1]
Allergy to local anesthetics	Sepsis or untreated bacteremia

Note: [1]Guidelines or consensus statements that address peripheral nerve blocks and anticoagulation or bleeding disorders have not been published at the time this book was written.

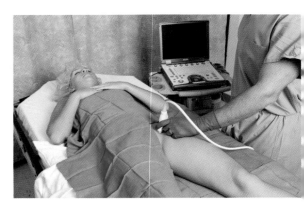

Figure 13.9 Proper set up and positioning for scanning for a femoral nerve block.

Table 13.4 Side effects and complications associated with femoral nerve block

Side effects	Complications
Motor blockade of quadriceps muscles for the duration of local anesthetic effect	

stomach. The ultrasound machine should be located near the head of the patient's bed, so that the screen is in an optimal viewing position for the physician, and the ultrasound controls are comfortably within the physician's reach. The physician performing the procedure should be positioned at the patient's surgical side with his/her body facing the patient and his/her head turned to see the ultrasound screen. The height of the bed should be adjusted so that the patient's

inguinal region is located in front of the physician's low- to mid-abdomen. The hand closest to the patient should control the ultrasound probe (Figure 13.10). A wide, sterile preparation is applied to the inguinal region, and sufficient ultrasound gel is applied to the site or probe to ensure adequate imaging.

The ultrasound probe is positioned along the *transverse* plane (Figures 13.10 and 13.11) near the inguinal crease, so that the orientation marker of the probe is positioned at the patient's *right* side. This will yield an ultrasound image in the transverse plane to the target structures. The depth of the scan and the position of the ultrasound probe should be adjusted (large movements) as needed in order to locate the pulsing femoral artery. This is the *orienting structure*, thus it should be the first structure identified when scanning for this procedure. Once this has been identified, the probe should be minimally tilted and

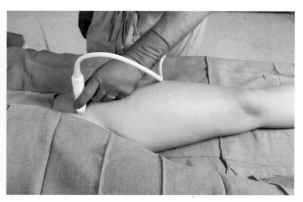

Figure 13.10 Proper ultrasound probe positioning for scanning at femoral region.

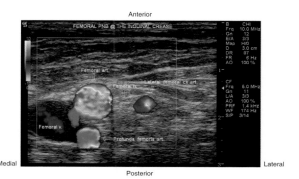

Figure 13.11 Color-flow showing both profunda femoris and lateral circumflex femoral arteries in the inguinal region.

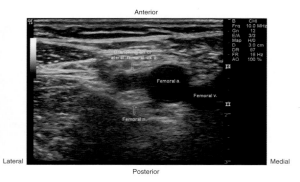

Figure 13.12 Branching of the lateral circumflex femoral artery off the femoral artery and crossing superficial to the femoral nerve.

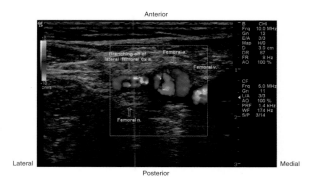

Figure 13.13 Same image as in Figure 13.12, shown with color-flow option to help verify hypoechoic structure as vascular.

rotated (small movements) in order to visualize a well defined, circular, cross-sectional view of the artery. Next, identify the femoral vein, which should be located just medial to the artery. Once both the femoral artery and vein have been identified, look for the *hyperechoic* femoral nerve located just lateral to the femoral artery (Figure 13.8).

At this point, we advise to complete scanning in the vicinity of the target structure to ensure that there is no unexpected anatomy (e.g., anomalous vessels) near the femoral nerve or along the anticipated path of the needle (from lateral). Next, perform a systematic scan slightly cephalad and caudad from the original scanning site to identify the proximity to the branching or location of the profunda femoris and lateral circumflex femoral arteries (Figure 13.12). Also, special attention should be paid to establish whether there is variant branching of the lateral circumflex femoral artery directly off the femoral artery (Figures 13.13 and 13.14).

Because of the proximity of these vascular structures to the femoral nerve, identify an area that is a comfortable distance from these structures to perform the nerve block. Without the use of ultrasound, vascular puncture can occur as high as 6% of the time when performing a femoral nerve block lateral to the femoral arterial pulse. Therefore, the precise location where these branches of the femoral artery occur, and their relative positions and proximity to the femoral nerve, is to be identified with the ultrasound in order to potentially minimize the chance of a vascular puncture.

Additional considerations

When performing the initial scan and having difficulty identifying the femoral vein, it may be due to the operator pressing too hard on the skin with the ultrasound probe. This may collapse the femoral vein and distort the overall anatomy.

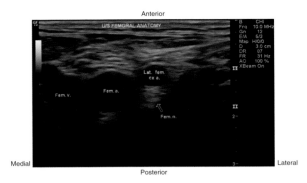

Figure 13.14 Image of a hypoechoic structure positioned superficial to the femoral nerve.

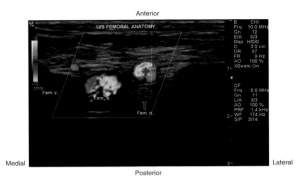

Figure 13.15 Same image as in Figure 13.14, with color-flow option to show that the hypoechoic structure is vascular.

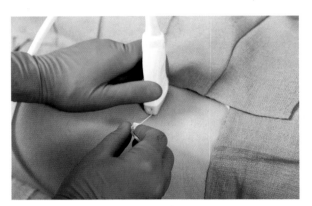

Figure 13.16 Ultrasound and in-plane needle positioning for performance of a femoral nerve block.

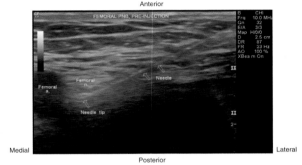

Figure 13.17 Proper initial needle position prior to local anesthetic injection.

The proximity of the femoral nerve to the femoral artery was one of the most surprising findings when we began performing ultrasound-guided femoral nerve blocks.

When uncertain as to whether a hypoechoic structure is vasculature (Figure 13.14), use the available functions on the ultrasound machine of either color-flow (Figure 13.15) and/or pulse-wave Doppler to help identify the structure in question

The diameter of the lateral circumflex femoral artery is usually one-third to half that of the femoral artery.

Needle insertion

Once an adequate image has been obtained and it has been deemed safe to perform the block, a skin wheal is raised with local anesthetic at the lateral end of the ultrasound probe. A blunt-tipped needle is placed through the wheal and advanced *in-plane* (IP) with the ultrasound beam in a lateral to medial direction, posteriorly towards the femoral nerve (Figure 13.16).

Look for the needle or movement in the upper corner (anterior-lateral) of the screen. Once the needle is under the transducer, it should become visible as a hyperechoic line. Do not blindly advance the needle. If the needle is not initially visible, stop and look at your hands to make sure that the needle is passing straight in the beam of the ultrasound probe. If it appears as though it should be but the needle remains not visible on the screen, you may need to make very small tilting or rotating movements with the probe to bring the needle into view. The initial image of your target structures should change very minimally, if at all. If the original scan has changed significantly in order to locate the needle, remove the needle and begin from the initial scanning step. The path of the needle should be aimed just lateral to the femoral nerve, then steering the needle around and posterior to the nerve. The ideal initial needle-tip placement before injection should be just posterior to the middle, or medial half, of the femoral nerve (Figure 13.17). Special care should be taken to avoid contacting the nerve, in order to minimize the potential for nerve damage.

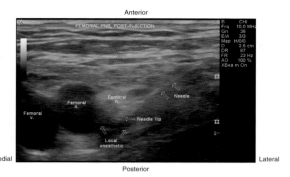

Figure 13.18 Injection through a properly positioned needle for a femoral nerve block.

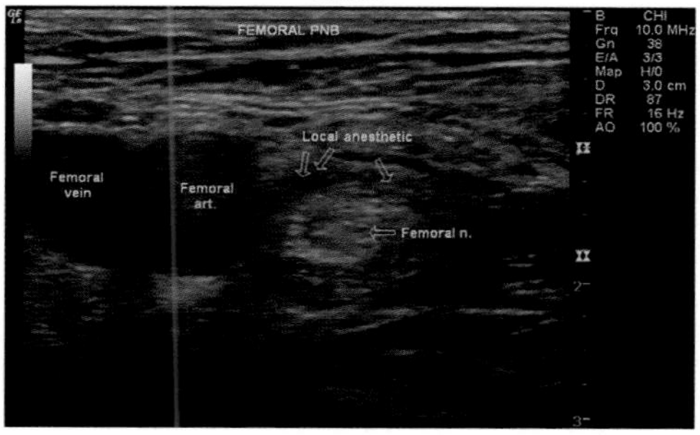

Figure 13.19 Post-injection femoral nerve block, with local anesthetic surrounding the nerve in a classic "donut sign".

Additional considerations

The most important part of the needle to keep in constant visualization is the needle tip. If the tip is not constantly visualized, it is difficult to be certain as to where it is located and what structures it may be penetrating. The only part of the needle that can be visualized is the part that is traveling through the narrow ultrasound beam.

Local anesthetic injection and needle repositioning

Once the needle is positioned in the ideal initial location, and initial negative aspiration of blood is confirmed, the injection of local anesthetic can begin (Figure 13.18). There should be frequent confirmation of negative aspiration after approximately every 3 to 5 ml of injection, and whenever the needle is repositioned. If there is high resistance to injection, stop and reposition the needle. Pay special attention to the spread of the local anesthetic, which will appear as an expanding hypoechoic region. It should be in a well contained space, not extending around the femoral vessels. The ideal spread should be circumferential around the femoral nerve yielding a "donut sign" in which the hyperechoic femoral nerve is floating in the middle of a hypoechoic circle of local anesthetic (Figure 13.19). If this circumferential spread of local anesthetic is not observed, reposition the needle, keeping the needle tip deep to the fascia lata, as needed in order to achieve the ideal local anesthetic spread. Make certain to reconfirm negative aspiration before injection every time the needle is repositioned.

Additional considerations

A negative aspiration does not rule out an intravascular injection.

Remain alert to the possibility of intravascular injection if the spread of local anesthetic is not seen, as this may indicate that the local anesthetic is being deposited into a vessel and not perineurally.

Take special care to avoid injection within the femoral nerve, which can be identified as a hypoechoic spread within the hyperechoic nerve with initial injection.

Stopping injection after every 3 to 5 ml to reconfirm negative aspiration of blood can help slow down the speed of injection, which can potentially decrease the pressure of injection.

Authors' clinical practice

- *Dosing regimen for knee procedures*: we typically use 20 ml of 0.2% to 0.5% ropivacaine. If preservation of motor function is important, such as early aggressive physical therapy, then using 0.2% ropivacaine may be the better concentration. However, if preservation of motor function during the first 24 hours after placement of the block is not a high priority, then the patient may benefit more from the more dense and longer duration of analgesia provided by a higher concentration of ropivacaine. The volume and dose of anesthetic used will be influenced by the patient, the patient's history and relevant comorbid conditions, and the spread of the local anesthetic.
- *Dosing regimen for hip procedures*: we typically use 30 ml of 0.2% to 0.5% ropivacaine. As discussed above, if preservation of motor function

is important, then 0.2% ropivacaine is the better concentration to use, but if motor function in the first postoperative day is not important, then 0.5% ropivacaine may provide more analgesia. The volume and dose of anesthetic used will be influenced by the patient, the patient's history and relevant comorbid conditions, and the spread of the local anesthetic.

- In order to have the highest success with postoperative pain relief for patients undergoing hip procedures, it is critical that the nerve block be placed as proximal in the thigh as possible, usually in the region between the inguinal crease and the inguinal ligament.
- Perhaps by ensuring that the entire volume of local anesthetic is deposited in the correct fascial plane under direct ultrasound visualization, and with a more proximal injection site when compared to a nerve stimulator femoral nerve block (see "3-in-1" block above), this may allow more cephalad spread of local anesthetic under the iliacus fascia to more reliably reach and anesthetize the lateral femoral cutaneous and obturator nerves.

- Although we advocate attempting to surround the nerve with local anesthetic, there are no studies to support that this will lead to a more rapid onset, longer duration, or higher success rates. Our advocacy is based on our own clinical experience and assumptions based on anatomy and physiology.
- When a primary anterior cruciate ligament (ACL) repair surgery is performed with an autograft, it is often harvested from the hamstring tendon of the semitendinosis muscle. This area falls within the distribution of the sciatic nerve, and patients perceive pain in the medial-posterior area of the knee. A sciatic nerve block can be done to cover this pain, but we have found that this pain is typically not

significant enough to warrant an additional nerve block. Typically, aggressive treatment with pain medication intraoperatively and in the post anesthesia care unit (PACU), to get "on top" of the pain is sufficient, and most patients require very little oral pain medication postoperatively for this harvest site.

- Also, if a patient is experiencing severe pain from the autograft harvest site after ACL repair not well controlled with pain medications, consider performing a proximal (e.g., subgluteal approach) sciatic nerve block. But consider the risk vs. benefit between pain control and eliminating all motor function to the operative leg.
- Patients receiving a femoral peripheral nerve block are at risk of falling throughout the duration of their block. Consideration and discussion of this fall risk should take place with the patient prior to sedation and placement of the nerve block.

Suggested reading

Fakuda H, Ashida M, Ishii R, Abe S, Ibukuro K. (2005). Anatomical variants of the lateral femoral circumflex artery: an angiographic study. *Surg Radiol Anat*, **27**(3):260–4.

Ito H, Shibata Y, Fujiwara Y, Komatsu T. (2008). Ultrasound-guided femoral nerve block. *Masui*, **57**(5):575–9.

Marhofer P, Schrogendorfer K, Koinig H., *et al.* (1997). Ultrasonographic guidance improves sensory block and onset time of three-in-one blocks. *Anesth Analg*, **85**(4):854–7.

Orebaugh S L. (2006). The femoral nerve and its relationship to the lateral circumflex femoral artery. *Anesth Analg*, **102**(6):1859–62.

Vazquez M T, Murillo J, Maranillo E, Parkin I, Sanudo J. (2007). Patterns of the circumflex femoral arteries revisited. *Clin Anat*, **20**(2):180–5.

Winnie A P, Ramamurthy S, Durrani Z. (1973). The inguinal paravascular technique of lumbar plexus anesthesia: the "3-in-1 block". *Anesth Analg*, **52**(6):989–96.

Chapter 14

Ultrasound-assisted ankle block

Introduction and specific anatomy

The ankle block involves a series of basic-level blocks targeting the five nerves around the ankle joint that provide innervation to the foot. This block approach is indicated for anesthesia or analgesia in podiatry cases where blockade of the distal leg and ankle joint may not be desired. Four of the target nerves (the superficial and deep peroneal nerves, the tibial nerve, and the sural nerve) are branches of the sciatic nerve. The saphenous nerve is the terminal extension of the femoral nerve.

Anatomically, the tibial nerve and deep peroneal nerve can be considered "deep" nerves relative to the superficial peroneal nerve, saphenous, and sural nerves, which have a more superficial orientation. Use of ultrasound guidance is helpful for specific placement of anesthetic around the two "deep nerves" in place of less specific fanning techniques. Field blocks of the remaining three superficial nerves are typically adequate to complete the "ankle" block.

The tibial nerve (posterior tibial nerve)

A terminal branch of the sciatic nerve, the tibial nerve courses through the lower leg behind the gastrocnemius muscle before entering the foot. The nerve runs behind the medial malleolus in the ankle, sandwiched between the posterior tibial vessels anteriorly and the flexor hallucis longus muscle and tendon posterolaterally. The nerve ultimately divides to form the medial and lateral plantar nerves supplying the plantar aspect of the foot as well as portions of the heel. (Figure 14.1)

The tibial nerve can be easily blocked at the ankle with ultrasound-guided assistance for procedures involving the plantar aspect of the foot and toes.

The deep peroneal nerve

The deep peroneal nerve (DPN) is a deep branch of the common peroneal nerve lying deep to the extensor

hallucis longus tendon and extensor digitorum longus tendon in the distal leg. The nerve is anterior to the tibia and interosseous membrane and typically situated lateral to the anterior tibial artery just above the ankle joint. The nerve ultimately branches in the dorsum of the foot with its medial branch supplying cutaneous innervation to the web space between the first and second toes, and a lateral branch providing motor innervation to the middle toes.

Like the tibial nerve, ultrasound-guided block of the DPN is easily accomplished and useful for procedures involving the hallux, or web-space between the first and second toes.

The superficial peroneal nerve

The superficial peroneal nerve (SPN) is a second branch of the common peroneal nerve. The SPN courses deep to the peroneal muscles of the lateral leg, becoming superficial at the leg's midpoint. At the level of the ankle, the nerve sends cutaneous branches anteriorly to the dorsum of the foot.

The sural nerve

The sural nerve typically forms around the middle or proximal leg from cutaneous branches of both the tibial and common peroneal nerves. The nerve travels distally along the lower lateral leg in deep fascia prior to becoming superficial and coursing around the posterior portion of the lateral malleolus. The sural nerve provides cutaneous innervation to a portion of the lateral foot and ankle.

The saphenous nerve

The saphenous nerve and its cutaneous branches are the terminal extension of the femoral nerve into the medial leg below the knee. In the distal leg, the nerve provides sensory innervation to portions of the medial ankle and foot.

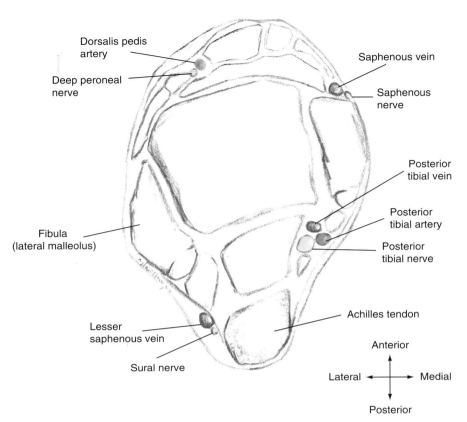

Figure 14.1 Cross-section of noting important structures ankle.

Ultrasound anatomy

Posterior tibial nerve

Orienting structure: the posterior tibial artery (Figure 14.2)

With the patient positioned supine, a high-frequency linear array probe is positioned behind the superior portion of the medial malleolus along the limb's short axis in order to create a transverse image of the nerves and vessels passing beneath the ultrasound beam (Figures 14.2 and 14.3).

Deep peroneal nerve

Orienting structure: the anterior tibial/dorsalis pedis artery (Figure 14.4)

With the patient supine, a high-frequency linear array probe is placed across the dorsal aspect of the patient's ankle joint along the limb's short axis to create a transverse image of the structures passing through the ultrasound beam. The DPN is

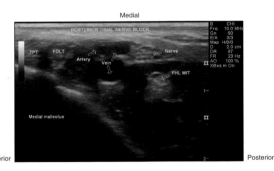

Figure 14.2 Transverse image of the structures behind the medial malleolus. Nerve = posterior tibial nerve; Vein = posterior tibial veins; TPT = tibialis posterior tendon; FDLT = flexor digitorum longus tendon; FHL M/T = flexor hallucis longus muscle/tendon.

typically oriented lateral to the vessels) (Figures 14.4 and 14.5).

Contraindications

Table 14.1 shows some contraindications to an ankle block.

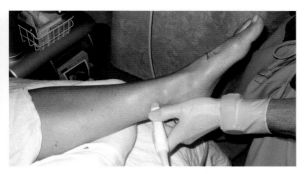

Figure 14.3 Positioning the ultrasound probe to image the posterior tibial nerve.

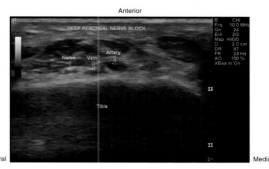

Figure 14.4 Deep peroneal nerve and dorsalis pedis artery and vein (right foot/ankle).

Structures that are required to be identified	Structures that may be seen
Posterior tibial vessels	Flexor digitorum longus tendon/muscle
Medial malleolus	Tibialis posterior tendon
	Flexor hallucis longus muscle/ tendon
	Calcaneal (Achilles) tendon

Side effects and complications

Table 14.2 shows some side effects and complications associated with an ankle block.

Equipment

- Ultrasound machine with high-frequency (10 to 15 MHz) linear array transducer
- Three or four 10-ml syringes with appropriate local anesthetic, equipped with 25-gage needles
- Sterile cover for ultrasound probe
- Sterile ultrasound gel
- Sterile gloves
- Appropriate sedation, monitoring, and oxygen supply
- Illustrated in Figure 14.6

Technique
Technique summary

1. Monitors placed and patient appropriately sedated
2. Sterile preparation applied to procedural site

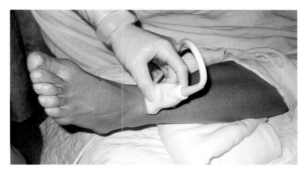

Figure 14.5 Ultrasound transducer placement for imaging the deep peroneal nerve.

Structures that are required to be identified	Structures that may be seen
Anterior tibial/dorsalis pedis vessels	Extensor hallucis longus tendon
Tibia	Extensor digitorum longus tendon

3. Sterile adhesive cover applied to ultrasound probe
4. Perform systematic ultrasound scan behind medial malleolus to find optimal location for placement of PTN block
5. Insert 25-gage block needle and guide toward target structures
6. Inject local anesthetic
7. Reposition needle as necessary to complete block
8. Repeat steps 4–7 for DPN ultrasound-guided nerve block
9. Perform remaining three field blocks to complete ankle block

The tibial nerve (posterior tibial nerve)

Scanning

With the patient positioned supine, the lower extremity to be blocked should be slightly elevated on blankets or a pillow with a small amount of external rotation at the hip to maximize exposure of the medial ankle. Using proper sterile technique, a high-frequency linear array transducer is positioned at the superoposterior border of the medial malleolus and oriented perpendicular to the leg. The target structures will be very superficial and the ultrasound depth setting should be adjusted appropriately. Obtain a

Table 14.1 Contraindications to ankle block

Absolute contraindications	Relative contraindications
Patient refusal	Contralateral neuromuscular disease/damage in ambulatory patient
Infection over site of needle insertion	
Allergy to local anesthetics	

Table 14.2 Side effects and complications associated with ankle block

Side effects	Complications[1]
Patient is at fall risk following block placement until block resolution	

Note: [1]Infection, nerve damage, local anesthetic toxicity, vascular injury, excessive bleeding, or hematoma are potential complications common to all nerve blocks.

tranverse image of the pulsatile posterior tibial artery, the orienting structure for this block. Use of the color-flow imaging function can sometimes be helpful (Figure 14.7a and b). It may be necessary to scan posterior toward the calcaneal tendon initially as well as proximally along the ankle to achieve the best image. The nerve typically appears posterior to the artery with mixed echogenicity (Figure 14.8).

Needle insertion

A 25-gage block needle is directed *in plane* with the starting position at the border of the malleolus. Observe advancement of the needle to a position *near* the target structure (Figures 14.9 and 14.10).

If the medial malleolus obstructs the path of the needle, follow the nerve above the malleolus to a more proximal position where the needle can be directed with less difficulty.

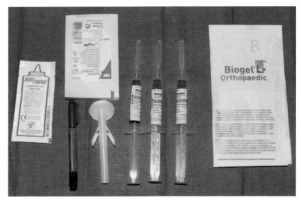

Figure 14.6 Equipment tray prepared for ultrasound-assisted ankle block.

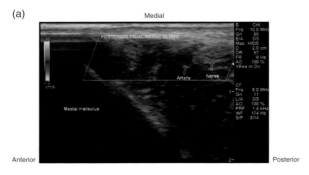

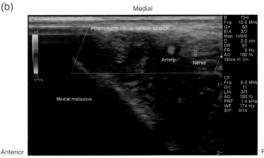

Figure 14.7 a and b Use of color-flow imaging to aid identification of the posterior tibial artery.

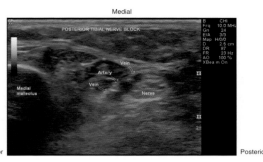

Figure14.8 Posterior tibial nerve and vessels. Nerve (arrow) is posterior to vessels.

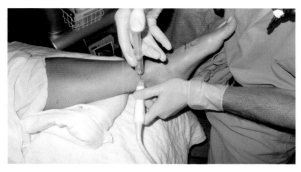

Figure 14.9 Needle insertion during posterior tibial nerve block.

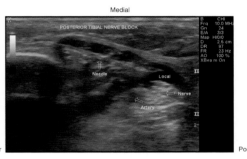

Figure 14.10 Needle positioning and local anesthetic injection around the posterior tibial nerve.

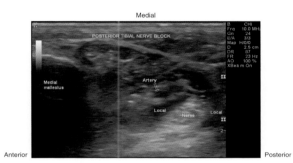

Figure 14.11 Completing a posterior tibial nerve block.

Additional considerations

Though the patient may be sedated he/she should be cooperative enough to hold the extremity still when the block is being placed. Surprising the sedated patient with a needle stick risks injury to the patient and physician performing the block. The patient's leg can be difficult to control by the sole practitioner when ultrasound guidance is utilized, and assistance from a nurse or second physician may be helpful.

Alternatively, a blunt bevel block needle may be used for the ultrasound-guided portions of the ankle block, with a local skin wheal placed at the site of needle insertion. This may give the operator more control with less risk for needle-stick injury during needle positioning.

An out-of-plane approach may also be used for this block. Using an out-of-plane approach will shorten the distance the needle must travel to the target. Be careful, however, (especially when approximating a sharp-tip needle near the nerve or neighboring blood vessels) as the needle trajectory is less easily identified using an out-of-plane approach.

Local anesthetic injection and needle repositioning

A total of 5 to 8 ml of local anesthetic should be injected around the nerve. The goal is to surround the nerve completely with anesthetic, and more than one pass with the block needle may be necessary in order for this to be accomplished (Figures 14.10 and 14.11).

The deep peroneal nerve
Scanning

The DPN is located in proximity to the dorsalis pedis artery. The nerve can be difficult to visualize under ultrasound guidance but is usually lateral to the vessels between the extensor hallucis and extensor digitorum longus tendons.

Following skin and transducer preparation, a high-frequency linear array transducer is oriented across the anterior aspect of the ankle at the level of the malleoli to generate a transverse image of the structures below. Note the appearance of the dorsalis pedis artery (orienting structure) and vein in cross-section just above the tibia. The nerve is small, and will be located adjacent to the vessels with hypo- or mixed echogenicity (Figure 14.12).

129

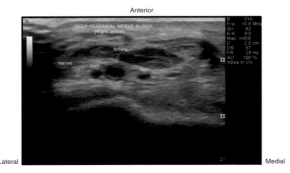

Figure 14.12 Deep peroneal nerve adjacent to dorsalis pedis artery and veins (right foot/ankle).

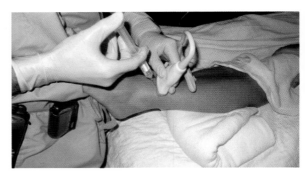

Figure 14.13 Needle insertion (out-of-plane approach) during deep peroneal nerve block.

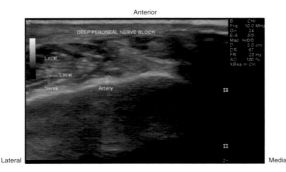

Figure 14.14 Local anesthetic injection around the deep peroneal nerve.

Needle insertion

Needle insertion is easily performed using an *out-of-plane* approach for this procedure due to the limited surface area on the anterior aspect of the ankle. A 25-gage block needle is directed toward the target structure from below the midpoint of the ultrasound transducer (Figure 14.13). Note the tissue displacement that occurs as the needle is advanced in order to help identify the tip's position. Steep angling of the block needle is required to direct the needle tip within the narrow ultrasound beam.

Additional considerations

Remember to warn the patient or control the extremity being blocked before needle insertion.

An in-plane approach to the DPN block is also feasible, and some practioners may be more comfortable advancing the needle in-plane from a lateral position along the anterior ankle.

Local anesthetic injection and needle repositioning

If the nerve is easily visualized, surround it with 3 to 5 ml of local anesthetic. The nerve may appear to float in the pool of anesthetic. If difficulty is encountered identifying the nerve, anesthetic may be injected adjacent to either side of the dorsalis pedis vessels as the nerve is typically in proximity (Figure 14.14).

The superficial peroneal nerve, sural nerve, and saphenous nerve

The remaining nerves involved in the ankle block provide cutaneous innervation to the foot and are easily blocked by a subcutaneous "ring", or field block, of local anesthetic around the ankle.

The SPN is blocked subcutaneously across the anterior aspect of the ankle connecting the proximal borders of the malleoli. Using the insertion point for the deep peroneal nerve, a field block can be carried first toward the medial aspect of the ankle and then the lateral. This leaves essentially one needle entry on the anterior aspect of the ankle. A total of 8 to 10 ml of local anesthetic is typically used (Figure 14.15).

The sural nerve is then blocked by continuing the SPN field block around the lateral aspect of the ankle toward the calcaneal tendon above the proximal aspect of the lateral malleolus (Figure 14.16). In similar fashion, the saphenous nerve is blocked on the medial ankle by injecting anesthetic subcutaneously from the proximal medial border of the medial malleolus to the calcaneal tendon (Figure 14.17). Five to 10 ml of local anesthetic are typically used for these field blocks respectively. When completed, a partial subcutaneous "ring" of local anesthetic has been created, encompassing the anterior, medial,

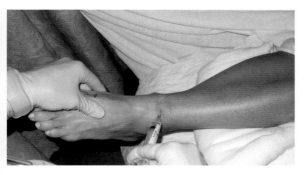

Figure 14.15 Superficial peroneal nerve field block.

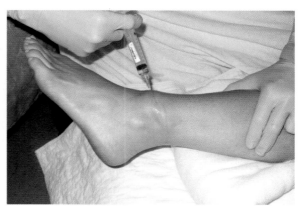

Figure 14.16 Sural nerve field block.

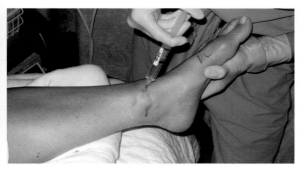

Figure 14.17 Saphenous nerve field block at the ankle.

and lateral portions of the ankle just proximal to the intermalleolar line.

Additional considerations

Ensure that a proper subcutaneous injection is completed. A superficial injection into the dermis of the skin can lead to block failure.

Attempt to minimize needle insertion points in order to reduce tissue trauma and discomfort for the patient.

Authors' clinical practice

- *Dosing regimen*: to maximize block duration and speed onset time we typically use 0.75% ropivacaine in divided doses: 5 to 8 ml for the posterior tibial nerve, 3 to 5 ml for the deep peroneal nerve, and 8 to 10 ml for each of the remaining three field blocks around the ankle.
- We often substitute 1.5% mepivacaine for shorter cases requiring surgical anesthesia without the need for extended postoperative analgesia.
- Ultrasound-guided placement of the posterior tibial and deep peroneal nerve blocks eliminates the need to use non-specific fanning techniques commonly used with these blocks. We find this has led to an increase in placement and success of these blocks in our practice.
- For beginners, use of ultrasound to complete this block may lengthen the time required for placement. With practice, however, this time discrepancy seems to diminish.

Suggested reading

Redborg K E, Antonakakis J G, Beach M L, Chinn C D, Sites B D. (2009). Ultrasound improves the success of a tibial nerve block at the ankle. *Reg Anesth Pain Med*, **34** (3):256–60.

Soares L G, Brull R, Chan V W. (2008). Teaching an old block a new trick: ultrasound-guided posterior tibial nerve block. *Acta Anaesthesiol Scand*, **52**(3):446–7.

Introduction to continuous perineural catheters

Introduction

Over the past several years, there has been an increasing interest and use in practice of continuous perineural catheters. The main area of focus has been their use in the management of acute postoperative pain following orthopedic procedures. Poorly controlled postoperative pain is one of the top reasons for delay of discharge of a patient from the post anesthesia care unit (PACU), or for the unexpected admission of a patient to the hospital. In addition, short-duration (e.g., single-injection peripheral nerve block, intra-articular injections) or ineffective postoperative pain control are important contributing factors that can lead to unanticipated readmission of patients to the hospital for pain management. With the ever-increasing shift to make more surgeries outpatient procedures, or to decrease the duration of a patient's hospital stay, a strong focus has been placed on developing strategies and techniques that can improve both the overall quality and duration of a patient's postoperative pain management. With the proper acute pain management set up and follow up, one can safely and effectively achieve this goal with the use of continuous perineural catheters for both inpatient and outpatient procedures.

Benefits of continuous perineural catheters

As more and more studies evaluate continuous peripheral nerve blocks (CPNB) and their role in postoperative pain control, more evidence is compiled to show their efficacy. Not only has the use of peri-neural catheters been shown to provide significantly better postoperative pain control than conventional therapy using parenteral or oral analgesics, the use of these catheters has also led to patients requiring dramatically less narcotic consumption. This has resulted in patients experiencing significantly fewer side effects associated with narcotic use, such as sedation, nausea, vomiting, and pruritis. In addition, patients who have had a CPNB experience better postoperative pain control when compared to patients who receive a single-injection peripheral nerve block without a catheter for similar procedures. More than just improving postoperative pain control, placement of a perineural catheter has been shown to improve the time to functional recovery during rehabilitation, as well as shorten the length of hospital stay for inpatient surgical procedures. With all of these advantages, it is not surprising that patients who receive a CPNB consistently report the highest satisfaction scores in regards to their postoperative analgesia.

Indications and selection criteria for perineural catheter placement

The decision as to which patient to offer a continuous perineural catheter is not always a clear one. Several factors must be examined:

First, certain *procedural factors* should be considered. A patient undergoing a more involved surgical procedure, such as a joint fusion or replacement, or a patient undergoing a less extensive surgical procedure that is known to be fairly painful postoperatively, such as shoulder surgery, could benefit from having a CPNB placed for postoperative analgesia. In addition to the specific surgery that is being performed, the postoperative physical therapy plan should also be considered. A patient who may not be undergoing an extensive procedure, but may be placed in a range-of-motion device for several days postoperatively, could benefit from the long-duration analgesia that a perineural catheter can offer. Also, aggressive physical therapy on postoperative Day 1 or earlier has become more and more common with orthopedic procedures. The placement of a continuous perineural catheter can aid in both the analgesia and time to functional recovery, which can improve the patient's rehabilitation.

133

Next, specific *patient factors* must be considered. Patients with a low pain tolerance, or a potential tolerance to pain medications as seen in some chronic pain patients, could benefit from a perineural catheter. This may be true even when the involvement of the surgery, or physical therapy plan, may not be significantly extensive. Also, there are some patients who may be highly sensitive to either the sedative or nauseating effects of narcotics and may wish to try more invasive techniques, like a CPNB, to avoid or minimize taking those medications postoperatively.

Just as there are certain *patient factors* that could encourage one to place a CPNB for a patient, regardless of the *procedural factors*, there are also *patient factors* that could discourage the placement of a CPNB. Some of these include:

- *Patient refusal*: not all patients are open to the idea of having an indwelling foreign body such as a perineural catheter. Since patient refusal is considered to be an absolute contraindication to a regional nerve block, this holds true for placement of a perineural catheter as well.
- *Patient understanding/communication*: some patients are just not capable of accepting the extra responsibility that comes with a perineural catheter and pump, especially when discharged home with them. It may be that the patient's cognitive abilities are not adequate enough to understand how to properly care for the pump and catheter site, or the patient may have significant psychiatric issues that may cloud the patient's reason or understanding. Sometimes the patient may not speak English well and, although they have the mental capability to understand the proper use and care of their pump and catheter as well as any potential follow up, this understanding may literally be lost in translation.
- *Geography*: if a patient lives significantly far away from the hospital or center where one practices, that patient may not be willing to return from home if any issues arise with the perineural catheter that need to be addressed in person. Since CPNBs are a relatively new procedure in the practice of anesthesia, and not universally performed, if the patient went to the local urgent care or emergency room to have the issue addressed, there is a good chance that the physician assessing the patient would not be familiar with perineural catheters. For this reason,

we make certain that the patient agrees to commit to return to our practice site in the rare situation that a catheter issue needs to be addressed in person before we consider placing a catheter in that patient.

- *Coagulation status*: since the needle used to place a perineural catheter is typically larger (17- or 18-gage) than the one used for a single-injection block, there is potentially more risk for vascular damage and hematoma if a vascular puncture occurs with the larger needle. For this reason one must first be comfortable with the patient's preoperative coagulation status prior to placing a CPNB, as well as the plan for postoperative coagulation status when the catheter is removed.
- *Patient cooperation/sedation ability*: again, the needle used to place a perineural catheter is typically larger (17- or 18-gage) than the one used for a single-injection block, so there is more potential for patient discomfort during or after catheter placement. Also, placing a perineural catheter takes significantly longer than placing a single-injection nerve block. These factors may negatively affect a patient's ability to cooperate during CPNB placement, so one must be prepared to potentially sedate the patient more heavily before placing the catheter than one might before placing a single-injection peripheral nerve block. For example, a highly anxious patient with significant obstructive sleep apnea may not be able to tolerate the level of sedation necessary to allow for the successful and sterile placement of a CPNB.
- *Postoperative infection risk*: patients with bacteremia or infection at or near the CPNB site are fairly obvious patients in whom to avoid placing an indwelling catheter. Other factors such as patients with poor personal hygiene, poorly controlled diabetes, or active/frequent illicit drug use may also raise concern for sterile maintenance of the CPNB site postoperatively. All of the considered factors should be amplified whenever any of these catheters are placed in patients who will be going home with the CPNB in place.

Infectious risk of perineural catheters

One of the major concerns before an anesthesiologist decides to begin placing perineural catheters in his or her practice is the infectious risk of the indwelling catheter. Several studies have examined this and found that the risk for infectious complications from CPNBs ranges from 0 to 3.2%, whereas the risk for severe infectious complications such as abscess formation requiring surgical drainage is low, ranging from 0 to 0.9%. Localized inflammation at the catheter insertion site can occur 0 to 4.3% of the time, but bacterial colonization of the catheter itself can occur anywhere from 0 to 57% of the time. If there is local inflammation or irritation at the catheter insertion site, there is a higher incidence of catheter bacterial colonization. The most frequently isolated microorganism identified on the colonized catheter is *Staphylococcus epidermidis*, which is also the most frequently isolated microorganism on the skin surface. However, the most frequently isolated microorganism reported in systemic infections or abscess formations associated with CPNBs is *Staphylococcus aureus*.

Several independent risk factors for development of catheter bacterial colonization and related infection have been identified: one of the most significant risk factors is a patient who spends time in the intensive care unit (ICU). Most of the patients that would fall into this category and still have a CPNB are likely to be victims of a major trauma. It has been suggested that the compromised cellular immunity that ICU patients typically experience, as well as the larger number of skin bacteria that trauma ICU patients tend to have, may play a role in this increased risk even when a strict aseptic technique is followed when placing a CPNB.

Another significant independent risk factor for the development of infection with CPNBs is the duration the catheter is in place. One study showed that keeping the perineural catheter in place for >48 hours is associated with increasing the risk of local inflammation and local infection, although only 1 case out of 1,416 (0.07%) developed a systemic infection. Other studies found that patients with no infections had a perineural catheter in place for an average of four days or less, while an average perineural catheter duration greater than four days was associated with a higher rate of infection requiring surgical drainage. Although there seems to be a relatively large and safe therapeutic window for the duration of keeping a CPNB in place, the longer the perineural catheter stays in place, the greater the risk of infection.

Other independent risk factors for potential infection with perineural catheters include male gender, absence of antibiotic prophylaxis, and site of catheter insertion. Femoral and axillary sites have a higher bacterial colonization rate than other sites, likely due to the larger density of sebaceous glands in these areas affecting the ability to disinfect properly.

In addition to being mindful of the independent risk factors when placing and managing CPNBs, one must follow the guidelines set by the American Society of Regional Anesthesia and Pain Medicine (ASRA) and adhere to a strict aseptic technique when placing these catheters. This includes hand washing, use of protective barriers (hat, mask, sterile gloves, gowns, and drapes) and skin disinfectants. Although povidine iodine and chlorhexidine gluconate are both considered appropriate, chlorhexidine does seem to have a distinct advantage over iodine. This is largely due to isopropyl alcohol in chlorhexidine giving more immediate bactericidal effects, as well as chlorhexidine's ability to adhere to the stratum corneum, which extends its duration of action for several hours after it has been applied.

Catheter placement and securing

Equipment

- Ultrasound machine
- Appropriate frequency ultrasound probe
- Mayo stand or bedside table
- Sterile gown, sterile gloves, hat, and mask
- Sterile skin preparation
- Sterile drape for the procedure site
- Sterile ultrasound controls cover (preferably clear)
- Sterile ultrasound probe sheath with two rubber bands
- Sterile ultrasound gel
- Sterile gauze
- Local anesthetic for skin and subcutaneous infiltration at block needle site insertion
- Blunt-tipped, large-gaged Tuohy needle of appropriate length (17-gaged needle needed to place 19-gage catheter; 18-gage needle needed to place 20-gage catheter)
- Appropriate local anesthetic and volume in sterile syringes
- Intravascular test dose containing epinephrine
- Sterile, *flexible* catheter with depth markers
- Catheter adapter for syringe/infusion tubing
- Strong skin adhesive, such as Dermabond® (Ethicon, Inc., Summerville, NJ, USA) or

Histoacryl® (B/BRAUN, Germany; TissueSeal, LLC, Ann Arbor, MI, USA), for securing catheter at insertion site

- Less strong adhesive, such as benzoin (Aplicare, Inc., Branford, CT, USA) or Mastisol® (Ferndale Laboratories, Inc., Ferndale, MI, USA) for securing clear dressing
- *Clear* Tegaderm™ (3M Health Care, St. Paul, MN, USA) dressing
- StatLock® (Venetec International, San Diego, CA, USA) or similar device
- Illustrated in Figure 15.1

Flexible perineural catheter: our experience has shown that the flexible catheters are more likely to coil within the fascial plane surrounding the nerve/plexus. The more rigid catheters tend to pop through this surrounding fascia, which positions the catheter tip away from the nerve/plexus and potentially penetrates into less ideal structures such as blood vessels, lung, muscle, or subcutaneous tissue.

Strong skin adhesive: in order to help stabilize the perineural catheter and minimize leakage of local anesthetic from the catheter insertion site we routinely apply either Dermabond® or Histoacryl® directly over where the catheter inserts into the skin. This should cover an area of approximately 1 to 2 cm around the catheter insertion site. Using this strong skin adhesive avoids the need to tunnel the catheter, minimizing the amount of times the integrity of the patient's skin is disrupted.

Less strong adhesive: spreading an agent like benzoin or Mastisol® over a larger area surrounding the catheter insertion site allows one to tightly coil the catheter on the skin, then securely place a clear, adhesive dressing over it all. This allows for a sterile dressing to be securely placed over the catheter site.

Clear dressing: it is important for this dressing to be clear, such as a Tegaderm™, because this allows the patient and/or caregiver to assess the catheter insertion site several times a day, watching for early signs of potential infection such as redness, inflammation, or pus.

StatLock®: this is a small plastic holder where the hub on the end of the catheter can be locked into place and adhered to the patient. It acts as further reinforcement to keep the catheter in place if any excessive tension pulls on it, like if a patient drops his/her pump or the catheter tubing gets tangled in

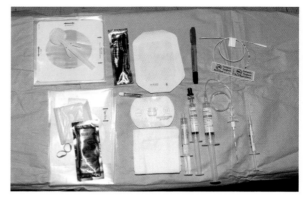

Figure 15.1 Layout of equipment for perineural catheter placement.

clothes or bed sheets. It also helps to prevent the hub from becoming detached from the catheter itself in any of these potential situations.

There are several perineural catheter kits on the market but, at the time of this publication, very few ultrasound-specific catheter kits exist, and the ones that exist we have found to be fairly incomplete. One may use an existing kit, ultrasound-specific catheter kit, or stimulating catheter kit, and simply grab the extra materials needed from one's stock area in order to perform the procedure. This may quickly become a tedious undertaking, though, if one's practice contains a moderate or high volume of potential perineural catheter placements. In this case one may work with a trusted vendor, as we did, to create a specialized ultrasound-specific perineural catheter kit that can fit the specific needs of you and your practice.

Set-up for unassisted catheter placement

Continuous perineural catheters should be placed under strict sterile technique with the physician and his/her assistant, when available, wearing a surgical cap, mask, sterile gown, and sterile gloves, as well as sterile covering of the ultrasound transducer and controls. When an assistant is not available, continuous perineural catheters can be placed by an unassisted anesthesiologist (Figure 15.2). In order to do this and maintain sterility of the equipment and the anesthesiologist, a number of steps must first take place to prepare the ultrasound machine, ultrasound probe, and catheter kit by the unassisted anesthesiologist. First, position the patient and place the ultrasound

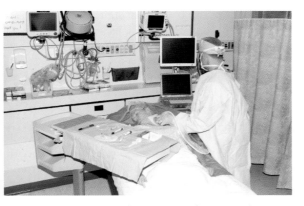

Figure 15.2 Proper set-up for placement of a perineural catheter by an unassisted anesthesiologist.

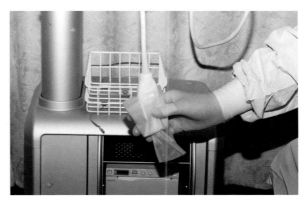

Figure 15.4 Sterile sheathing of an ultrasound probe.

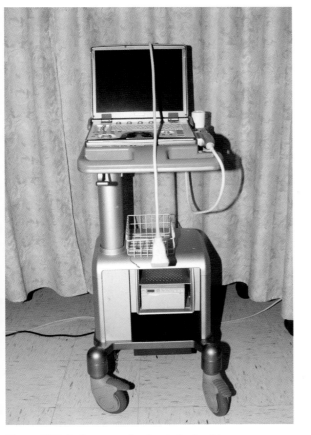

Figure 15.3 Probe preparation for sterile sheathing.

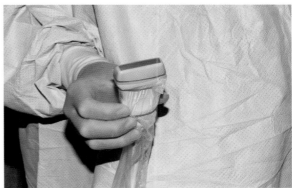

Figure 15.5 Even spread of ultrasound gel over the probe with the ultrasound probe sheath secured by two rubber bands.

machine at or near the head of the patient's bed, as in the single-injection technique. The ultrasound probe should then be draped over the front of the ultrasound machine, hanging freely (Figure 15.3). Next a block table with the equipment for placing the perineural catheter, sterilely laid out on it, is placed across the patient from the opposite side on which the block will be performed. At this point the anesthesiologist should don the cap, mask, sterile gown, and gloves. Next, a wide sterile preparation should be applied to the procedure site, followed by the placement of a clear, sterile drape over that area. Conduction gel should then be placed inside the sterile ultrasound probe sheath and the sheath then carefully placed over the hanging probe and draped over the cord (Figure 15.4). It is important that the gel be distributed evenly across the tip of the probe to ensure that there are no air bubbles between the probe and the sheath. A rubber band should then be placed across the top of the probe to maintain a snug fit. A second rubber band should then be applied lower on the probe to ensure that the sheath does not slide while the probe is being handled (Figure 15.5). Once the probe is covered, the ultrasound machine

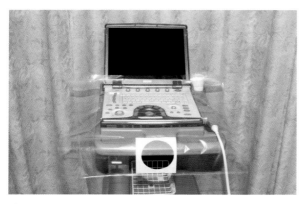

Figure 15.6 Clear sterile drape over the ultrasound controls.

controls should be draped with a clear, sterile cover (Figure 15.6). Lastly, a small amount of the remaining conduction gel should be placed on the patient, so that scanning and placement of the perineural catheter can now begin.

Infusion pump selection

When beginning evaluation of the many infusion pumps available on the market, several factors must be taken into consideration. First, there is no right or wrong infusion pump device, just what is best for you and your practice. To decide this, one must consider what needs are most important to one's continuous peripheral nerve block (CPNB) service, then choose a pump that has the most characteristics to support those needs. These pump attributes include the following.

- *Reliability of function*: reliability will be defined as the expectation that the pump will function and continue to deliver a basal infusion rate and patient-controlled analgesia (PCA) capability, if one is available on the pump. It has been our experience that the elastomeric pumps have been more reliable than electronic pumps.
- *Accuracy of the infusion rate*: accuracy will be defined as the ability of the pump to infuse solution at the set rate, and its consistency to do so throughout the extent of the infusion. In general, the electronic pumps tend to be more accurate than elastomeric pumps. Also of note is that the infusion rates of elastomeric pumps may be decreased if one practices in hypobaric conditions, as can occur at high altitudes.
- *Patient-controlled analgesia*: whether or not the pump has a PCA bolus capability, and the options

in the dose and programmability of the PCA are important to consider. The use of a PCA on a CPNB pump, in addition to a basal infusion, has been shown to improve pain control for patients. Thus the inclusion of a PCA capability can be a useful trait for a pump, although it does add more complexity, which may affect the reliability of the pump. One can choose a pump in which the dose and time frame for the PCA can be individually programmed. This allows for specific alterations to the PCA dose and/or timing from one patient to the next. One may also choose a pump with a set PCA dose for a specific time frame, so that when one orders the pump, the PCA function has already been built in without the capability of altering it. The former PCA traits tend to be found with electronic pumps, where the latter traits are more typically found with elastomeric pumps. Like anything else, there are advantages and disadvantages with each. With the more specific PCA programmability pumps, the higher specificity allows for a more individualized treatment, but allows more potential for malfunction or error, including human error, which may affect the overall reliability of the pump's function. The less specific, predetermined PCA dose and timing pumps allow less room for individualizing treatment, but do minimize the potential for error and may affect pump reliability less.

- *Total local anesthetic volume capacity*: the total volume that the pump can hold will often dictate how long the CPNB will last. This is more important, though, if one's practice is likely to have outpatient perineural catheters because one cannot change or refill those pumps as easily as one can for inpatients. Most perineural catheters are meant to stay in and work for at least two days. Based on the basal infusion rate, and the PCA dose and frequency, one can often approximate how much volume would be ideal in order for the CPNB to last near the goal duration. Many pumps have a target fill volume but some can be overfilled, sometimes by a significant volume, and may result in up to a 10% change in the accuracy of the basal infusion rate.
- *Portability of the pump*: most pumps are relatively small and weigh less than a few pounds when filled with local anesthetic. These pumps should come with small carrying bags, with adjustable

straps, so that the patient can carry the pump comfortably in the bag. When pumps hold a large volume (e.g., overfilled), have an added PCA function or have a large electronic programming section, the pump unit may be larger and/or heavier, which may negatively affect its portability.

- *Ease of use and understanding*: the ease of use and understanding of the pump by both the anesthesiologist and the patient are very important. For the anesthesiologist, the spectrum of the ease of pump use may range from hooking it up and unclamping the tubing, to clearing histories and programming every aspect of the pump's set up and use. As long as all of the anesthesiologists in the group who will be placing and managing the CPNBs feel consistently comfortable with every aspect of the set up and programming of the pump, then this is likely of little concern. What is important, though, is that the patient be able to use the pump consistently well. From our experience, we have found that the less the patient needs to do, the better success they will have with the pump. The best scenarios have been once the pump has been reliably set up and attached to the perineural catheter, the patient should be expected to do very little with the pump outside of tote it with him/her and perhaps hit the PCA button as needed.

- *Disposability vs. reusability of the pump*: the disposability of the pump is often dictated by the patient. If one is placing the CPNBs exclusively for inpatients, perhaps a reusable, non-disposable pump would be best. If one's practice expects to place CPNBs in outpatients, perhaps a disposable pump would be more advantageous. This would be especially important when one's outpatient service does not require that the patient return in order to have the catheter removed.

- *Cost of the pump*: one must consider more than just the initial cost of the pump. If it is a reusable pump, one should consider the potential lifespan of the pump and potential service costs. Also, one should consider the potential for growth of the CPNB service and the future cost that may be associated with purchasing more reusable pumps. With disposable pumps, one should consider how long the pump may last relative to the cost of the pump. This will be dependent on the total volume capacity of the pump, including overfill capability, the planned infusion rate, whether or

not a PCA function will be used and the volume/frequency of it, and the refill capability of the pump and the associated costs.

The perfect pump may not exist, but one can decide the needs that are most important to the CPNB service and choose the pump with the most characteristics to support those needs.

Infusion and dosing regimen selection

Once an infusion pump has been selected, the next step involves deciding on the type of medication to infuse through the perineural catheter. Many local anesthetics of both short and long duration have been studied, but there have not been significant enough findings to determine which medication is best for use in CPNBs, especially when considering the ambulatory population. The majority of studies performed, though, have involved the longer acting local anesthetics such as ropivacaine, bupivacaine, and levobupivacaine. When comparing ropivacaine to bupivacaine at equal analgesic concentrations, ropivacaine was found to cause a less profound motor blockade. There were no significant differences when comparing equal analgesic concentrations of ropivacaine with levobupivacaine, though. Ropivacaine, typically at a concentration of 0.2%, appears to be a popular choice of CPNB infusate currently, especially when used in an ambulatory population. This may be in part due to a combination of its relatively safer local anesthetic toxicity profile, its relatively decreased motor blockade, and its comparable cost at this time. Studies investigating the inclusion of additives such as clonidine, narcotics, or epinephrine to the long-acting local anesthetic infusions have not shown any consistent benefit when compared to an infusion of only local anesthetic at this time.

Next, one must decide on what rate to infuse the local anesthetic, and whether or not to include a PCA function. Many investigations have attempted to find the optimal dosing regimen for CPNBs, but several factors affect the results. Variables such as the anatomic site of the perineural catheter (e.g., interscalene vs. infraclavicular vs. femoral, etc.), inpatients vs. ambulatory patients, specific local anesthetic infused, surgical procedure, and postoperative physical therapy plan can all affect the CPNB infusion regimen. One finding that has been shown to be consistently reproducible, though, is that providing a regimen that incorporates both a basal infusion with PCA boluses is superior in analgesia, decreasing narcotic consumption and sleep disturbances, and increasing patient satisfaction, when compared to using only a basal infusion rate or only a PCA function. This is especially true after procedures are performed that can cause moderate to severe postoperative pain. In addition, some investigations also found that the basal infusion rate may often be decreased when a PCA bolus is added to the regimen. Also, serum concentrations of local anesthetics in patients with no liver or renal disease have been shown to be within acceptable levels during CPNB infusions several days in duration. All this said, there is still no best dosing regimen for CPNBs. Successful CPNBs have been reported with basal infusions of 5 to 10 ml/hr, with PCA boluses of 2 to 5 ml every 20 to 60 minutes.

Discharge instructions and follow-up care

For any perineural catheter service, whether it is for inpatients, outpatients, or both, there must be a plan for the care of these patients once they leave the post anesthesia care unit (PACU). This typically involves providing patients with detailed education regarding their CPNB and pumps, a plan for follow-up care with the patients, and a catheter removal and pump return/disposal plan.

Patient education

Whether the patient is discharged home or transferred to a hospital room, we recommend that the patient receives instructions and education regarding the CPNB and pump prior to leaving the PACU. This can be performed by either an anesthesiologist or a trained and educated regional anesthesia or acute pain nurse. Whenever the patient is discharged home, whether it is from the PACU or from a hospital room, we recommend that the patient and a caretaker for that patient be educated at the same time, since the patient's cognitive ability may often be affected by the medications he/she has received. This education should involve both written and verbal instructions on proper post-discharge care and management of the CPNB. Our typical discharge instructions include, but are not limited to, the following:

- general information about what a CPNB is and how it works
- basic information on the pump, what it is filled with, how long it will last, and how to tell when it is empty

- care and monitoring of the perineural catheter site and dressing
- care of the pump
- common side effects that may occur with the specific CPNB the patient received
- weight-bearing instructions, if applicable
- how to assess, and what to do, if there is leaking at the perineural catheter site
- examples of reasons to call the anesthesiologist
- how to remove the perineural catheter and assess that the entire catheter has been removed
- how to dispose of the perineural catheter and pump
- contact number for CPNB pager.

Patient follow-up

The optimal frequency at which to follow up with patients depends on several factors such as whether it is an inpatient or an outpatient, the surgical procedure performed on the patient, any comorbidities the patient may have, and the amount of post-procedure management that the patient's CPNB may have required. It may be worthwhile to document not only the inpatient follow up, but the ambulatory patient contacts as well. For inpatients, we typically follow up with them at least once a day until the perineural catheter has been removed. For outpatients, broad ranges of follow-up care have been described. These can include contact by telephone in varying frequencies, home nursing visits, having the patients return to the surgical center for follow-up, or combinations of these. Also, it is often recommended that there be a contact number to call, or a plan in place for the patient to follow, if the patient has any concerns or complications that may arise from the CPNB. We typically contact our ambulatory patients by telephone at least once on their first postoperative day, and more frequently as needed. Also, the outpatients are given a contact telephone number to a pager that exists solely for patients who have been discharged with CPNBs. This pager is carried by the on-call anesthesiologist at all times. Patients are instructed to call this number with any significant question or concern regarding their CPNB throughout the duration of its infusion or after its removal.

Catheter removal and pump disposal/return

There are several different manners in which a perineural catheter can be removed. For inpatients, the catheters can be removed by either an anesthesiologist or a properly trained and educated nurse, whether it is a nurse from the patient's ward, a nurse anesthetist, or a specific regional anesthesia or acute pain nurse. Where more of the concern occurs is the proper manner in which to remove the perineural catheters in the ambulatory population. Several methods have been proposed that cover a broad range of care. One involves discharging the patients with written and verbal instructions on how they or their caretaker can remove the catheter at home. Another method involves removal of the catheter by the patient or their caretaker while receiving instructions via telephone from an anesthesiologist or trained nurse. The final method involves the patient returning to the surgical center, or another predetermined healthcare site, for removal of the perineural catheter by an appropriate healthcare provider. All of these have been evaluated and no one technique has been found to be superior. The method that is chosen to be implemented into practice will depend on available resources and comfort level with it. If instructions are given for the patient to remove the catheter at home, the patient should have immediate access to an anesthesiologist. In our practice, we provide very detailed verbal and written instructions to the patient and caretaker describing how either one of them can safely and cleanly remove the catheter at home. We further reinforce this and verify his/her understanding of these instructions during our first postoperative follow-up telephone call. The written discharge instructions contain the number to our CPNB pager, which is carried by the on-call anesthesiologist, so they have immediate access to us at any time.

Authors' clinical practice

- Leaking at the catheter site was the most common reason we were contacted by patients who were discharged home with perineural catheters. Since we began routinely applying strong skin adhesives, such as Dermabond® or Histoacryl®, to the catheter insertion site, there has been significantly reduced leakage, and now leaking at the catheter site is a very rare occurrence. This has led to

higher patient, as well as on-call anesthesiologist, satisfaction.

- If a practice has a significant volume of both in- and outpatient catheters, we recommend consolidating to the use of one pump, rather than two separate pumps. Two pumps produce more potential issues ranging from purchasing and filling of the pumps to confusing the nursing staff in the PACU and the floors (outpatients can sometimes spend the night in-house as 24-hr observation).

- When consolidating to one pump, we recommend choosing the pump that best suits the needs of the outpatient CPNBs. Any issues that may arise on the inpatients can typically be more easily and quickly dealt with than when the patient has already been discharged home. For this reason, we feel the characteristics that best fit the needs for outpatient CPNBs outweigh those for inpatient CPNBs.

- In our practice, we primarily use ropivacaine as our local anesthetic for CPNB infusions. Although our ropivacaine concentration and basal infusion rates change according to the site of our catheter, the surgical procedure for which it is placed, and the postoperative physical therapy plan, we typically run a relatively high basal infusion rate (8 to 10 ml/hr) with a PCA bolus of 2 to 5 ml every 30 minutes.

Suggested reading

De Ruyter M L, Brueilly K E, Harrison B A, et al. (2006). A pilot study on continuous perineural catheter for analgesia after total knee arthroplasty: the effect on physical rehabilitation and outcomes. *J Arthroplasty*, **21**(8):1111–17.

Grossi P, Allegri M. (2005). Continuous peripheral nerve blocks: state of the art. *Curr Opin Anaesthesiol*, **18**(5):522–6.

Ilfeld B M, Morey T E, Enneking F K. (2002). Continuous infraclavicular brachial plexus block for postoperative pain control at home: a randomized, double-blinded, placebo-controlled study. *Anesthesiology*, **96**(6):1297–304.

Ilfeld B M, Morey T E, Wang R D, Enneking F K. (2002). Continuous popliteal sciatic nerve block postoperative pain control at home: a randomized, double-blinded, placebo-controlled study. *Anesthesiology*, **97**(4):959–65.

Ilfeld B M, Morey T E, Wright T W, et al. (2003). Continuous interscalene brachial plexus block for postoperative pain control at home: a randomized, double-blinded, placebo-controlled study. *Anesth Analg*, **96**(4):1089–95.

Ilfeld B M, Thannikary L J, Morey T E, *et al.* (2004). Popliteal sciatic perineural local anesthetic infusion: a comparison of three dosing regimens for postoperative analgesia. *Anesthesiology*, **101**(4):970–7.

Ilfeld B M, Torey T E, Enneking F K. (2004). Infraclavicular perineural local anesthetic infusion: a comparison of three dosing regimens for postoperative analgesia. *Anesthesiology*, **100**(2):395–402.

Kaloul I, Guay J, Cote C, *et al.* (2004). Ropivacaine plasma concentrations are similar during continuous lumbar plexus blockade using the anterior three-in-one and the posterior psoas compartment techniques. *Can J Anaesth*, **51**(1):52–6.

Macaire P, Gaertner E, Capdevila X. (2001). Continuous post-operative regional anesthesia at home. *Minerva Anestesiol*, **67**(9 Suppl 1):109–16.

Mizuuchi M, Yamakage M, Iwasaki S, *et al.* (2003). The infusion rate of most disposable, non-electric infusion pumps decreases under hypobaric conditions. *Can J Anaesth*, **50**(7):657–62.

Richmond J M, Liu S S, Courpass G, *et al.* (2006). Does continuous peripheral nerve block provide superior pain control to opioids? A meta-analysis. *Anesth Analg*, **102**(1):248–57.

Swenson J D, Bay N, Loose E, *et al.* (2006). Outpatient management of continuous peripheral nerve catheters placed using ultrasound guidance: an experience in 620 patients. *Anesth Analg*, **103**(6):1436–43.

White P F, Issioui T, Skrivanek G D, *et al.* (2003). The use of continuous popliteal sciatic nerve block after surgery involving the foot and ankle: does it improve the quality of recovery? *Anesth Analg*, **97**(5):1303–9.

Chapter 16

Interscalene continuous perineural catheter

Introduction

Continuous interscalene catheters provide excellent postoperative analgesia for patients undergoing shoulder and proximal humerus surgery and can be used to prolong the duration of analgesia beyond that of a single-injection technique. Continuous catheter placement is considered an advanced technique and it is assumed that the physician has mastered the single-injection interscalene technique; therefore a detailed discussion on how to perform an interscalene nerve block is not included in this chapter.

Ultrasound anatomy review

Orienting structure: carotid artery (Figure 16.1)

Structures that are required to be identified	Structures that may be seen
Carotid artery	Transverse process
Internal jugular vein	Thyroid
Sternocleidomastoid muscle	Trachea
Anterior scalene muscle	Vertebral artery
Middle scalene muscle	
Trunks/divisions of the brachial plexus	
Deep cervical fascia	
Subclavian artery	
First rib/pleura	

Equipment

- Ultrasound machine
- High-frequency linear array ultrasound probe
- Mayo stand or bedside table
- Sterile gown, sterile gloves, hat, and mask
- Sterile skin preparation
- Sterile drape for the procedure site

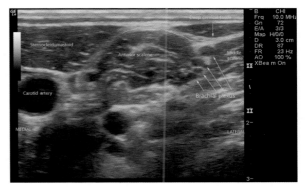

Figure 16.1 Ultrasound anatomy for an interscalene block with the carotid artery as the orienting structure.

- Sterile ultrasound machine controls cover (preferably clear)
- Sterile ultrasound probe sheath with two rubber bands
- Sterile ultrasound conduction gel
- Local anesthetic for skin and subcutaneous infiltration at block needle insertion site
- Blunt-tipped, large-gaged, 4-cm Tuohy needle (17-gage needle needed to place 19-gage catheter; 18-gage needle needed to place 20-gage catheter)
- Local anesthetic in 10-ml and 20-ml syringes
- Intravascular test dose containing epinephrine
- Sterile, *flexible* catheter with depth markers
- Catheter adapter for syringe/infusion tubing
- Strong skin adhesive (Dermabond® or Histoacryl®) for securing catheter at insertion site
- Less strong adhesive (benzoin or Mastisol®) for securing clear dressing
- *Clear* Tegaderm™ or OpSite™ dressing
- StatLock®
- Illustration in Figure 16.2

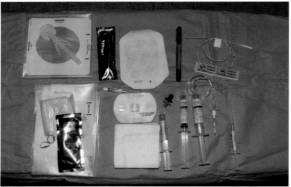

Figure 16.2 Ultrasound-guided perineural catheter kit contents.

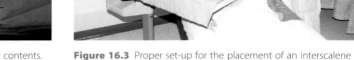

Figure 16.3 Proper set-up for the placement of an interscalene perineural catheter by an unassisted anesthesiologist.

Technique

Technique summary

1. Monitors placed and patient is appropriately sedated
2. Sterile preparation and drape to procedural site
3. Ultrasound probe and machine are sterilely draped
4. Perform systematic ultrasound scan to find optimal location for catheter insertion
5. Skin wheal is raised
6. Insert Tuohy needle and inject 20 ml of local anesthetic
7. Disconnect tubing from Tuohy needle
8. Insert catheter through Tuohy needle
9. Remove Tuohy needle while catheter held in place
10. Locate catheter on ultrasound image, then incrementally inject 10 ml of local anesthetic through catheter
11. Pull back on catheter as needed to optimize its position
12. Inject test dose containing epinephrine through catheter
13. Catheter insertion site is sealed with strong skin adhesive
14. Catheter is coiled and covered with benzoin and a Tegaderm™
15. Catheter hub is secured to the patient with a StatLock®

Patient and equipment preparation

Since continuous catheters require more time to place than single-injection nerve blocks, require the use of larger gage needles, and the patient's face is often covered with a sterile drape, this procedure may be more uncomfortable and anxiety provoking for the patient. Use of adequate sedation and an assistant, when possible, to monitor the patient and ensure that the patient does not reach into the procedural area and contaminate the field may be beneficial.

Continuous perineural catheters should be placed under strict sterile technique with the physician and his/her assistant, when available, wearing a surgical cap, mask, sterile gown, and sterile gloves, as well as sterile covering of the ultrasound transducer and controls. When an assistant is not available, continuous perineural catheters can be placed by an unassisted anesthesiologist (Figure 16.3). The steps taken to prepare the ultrasound machine, probe, and catheter kit by an unassisted anesthesiologist are as follows.

1. Position the patient and place the ultrasound machine at the head of the patient's bed, as in the single-injection technique, then drape the ultrasound probe over the front of the ultrasound machine, hanging freely (see Figure 15.3).
2. A block table with the equipment for placing a catheter, sterilely laid out on it, is placed across the patient from the opposite side on which the block is will be performed (see Figure 16.3).
3. The anesthesiologist should now don the cap, mask, and sterile gown and gloves.
4. Apply a wide sterile preparation to the neck and supraclavicular regions, then place a clear, sterile drape over the area.
5. Conduction gel is then placed inside of the sterile ultrasound probe sheath and the sheath is carefully placed over the hanging probe, then extended over the cord (see Figure 15.4). It is important that the gel is distributed evenly across the tip of the probe and

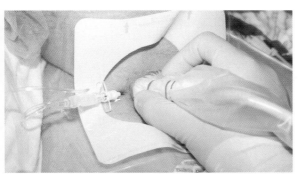

Figure 16.4 In-plane needle insertion: the needle is inserted away from the probe with a shallow needle-insertion angle.

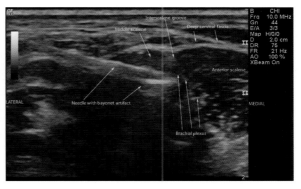

Figure 16.5 Tuohy needle positioned near the superior trunk of the brachial plexus: note the shallow angle of insertion.

to ensure that there are no air bubbles between the probe and the sheath. A rubber band is then placed across the top of the probe to maintain a snug fit. A second rubber band is then applied lower on the probe to ensure that the sheath does not slide while the probe is being handled (see Figure 15.5).

6. With the probe now covered, the ultrasound machine controls are draped with a clear, sterile cover (see Figure 15.6).

7. A small amount of the remaining sterile conduction gel is placed on the patient, so that scanning can now begin.

> **Additional considerations**
>
> Excessive amounts of conduction gel on the patient can make needle and catheter handling very difficult. Only use a minimal amount of conduction gel on the patient.

Scanning

Scanning for perineural catheters is carried out in the same way as for a single-injection interscalene brachial plexus block. However, the optimal location for the placement of a catheter may be different than that for a single-injection interscalene block. The placement of the catheter tip needs to be very precise. Higher concentrations and large volumes of local anesthetic used in single-injection blocks can overcome a less precise needle placement. Large volumes can (1) spread and block all three trunks of the brachial pleuxus when there is great separation between the trunks; (2) travel retrograde to block the roots of the brachial plexus and the superficial cervical plexus; and/or (3) block a suprascapular nerve that has branched from the superior trunk when the injection

is too caudal on the neck. If the catheter placement is not very precise, the infusion of local anesthetic from the catheter tip may not reach all the structures reached by the initial large bolus of local anesthetic.

Strive to place the catheter tip between the superior and middle trunks of the brachial plexus as far cephalad on the neck as possible. Scan to find a location with good ultrasound visualization of the superior and middle trunks. Cephalad placement of the catheter will increase the likelihood of local anesthetic traveling retrograde to block the roots of the brachial plexus and the superficial cervical plexus. A cephalad location should also increase the probability of blocking the suprascapular nerve.

> **Additional considerations**
>
> Aim for as cephalad a needle insertion as possible for shoulder surgery.

Needle insertion

The Tuohy needle is inserted in plane, as in a single-injection interscalene block, and advanced under ultrasound visualization towards the brachial plexus. The goal is to position the tip of the needle near the superior and middle trunks of the brachial plexus. Avoid contacting the brachial plexus and do not advance the needle through the brachial plexus.

Needle insertion should be away from the edge of the probe, not right next to the probe (Figure 16.4). Inserting the needle away from the probe forces the catheter to travel further before reaching the brachial plexus, as well as forcing the use of a shallow needle-insertion angle to reach the brachial plexus (Figure 16.5). Recall that a

145

shallow needle-insertion angle to the probe will make needle visualization easier. Due to their larger diameter, needles used to place catheters may be visualized even with relatively steep needle-insertion angles. However, a shallow needle-insertion angle is still recommended in order to help secure the catheter and better visualize the catheter once the needle is removed.

Due to the superficial location of the brachial plexus in the interscalene region, and the lack of a large muscle to anchor the catheter as it passes through to the brachial plexus, only a few centimeters of the catheter may be secured in subcutaneous tissue and muscle, especially in thin patients; this may increase the risk of catheter movement and dislodgement. Using a shallow insertion angle forces the needle, and therefore the catheter, to travel a greater distance in tissue before reaching the target, which may help stabilize the catheter.

Insertion of a perineural catheter requires the use of a large-bore needle, relative to the needle used for placement of a single-injection block. The number of needle passes made should be kept to a minimum, as these large, blunt needles are capable of considerable tissue trauma. Multiple passes may lead to bruising, pain, and tears of arteries and veins. These large, blunt needles can also create channels that allow leakage of local anesthetic after catheter placement. The deep cervical fascia can act as a barrier to keep local anesthetic from leaking. If multiple needle passes are required, redirect the needle with the tip beneath the deep cervical fascia to minimize the number of punctures in this fascia. Leakage of local anesthetic is problematic for several reasons, as follows.

- Local anesthetic leakage away from the brachial plexus decreases the volume of local anesthetic around the brachial plexus and may lead to catheter failure and patient discomfort.
- Wetness from leaking local anesthetic may undo the dressing placed over the catheter insertion site, which may increase the likelihood of catheter dislodgement.
- Wetness at the dressing and dripping of local anesthetic is very uncomfortable for patients and may cause requests for early discontinuation of the catheter by the patient.

Additional considerations

The most important part of the needle to keep in constant visualization is the needle tip. If the tip is not constantly visualized, one is never certain as

to where it is located and what structures it may be penetrating. The only part of the needle that can be visualized is the part that is traveling through the narrow ultrasound beam.

Do not touch the brachial plexus trunks with the Tuohy needle.

Large Tuohy needles may give a bayonet artifact during this block.

Local anesthetic injection and needle repositioning

With the Tuohy needle positioned near the superior and middle trunks of the brachial plexus, injection of local anesthetic can be carried out (Figure 16.6). Observe the pattern of spread to confirm positioning of the needle tip within the correct fascial plane. The needle can be repositioned if spread of local anesthetic is not within the correct fascial plane. Remember to keep needle movements small and the tip below the deep cervical fascia. Injection through the Tuohy needle prior to placement of the catheter serves several purposes, as follows.

- Injection of local anesthetic, and observance of the spread, serves as a confirmation as to the location of the needle tip within the correct fascial plane so that the catheter will also be in the correct fascial plane.
- Local anesthetic injection can expand the surrounding tissue and make passage of the catheter easier.
- If the catheter is not positioned in the proper location initially, by injecting some local anesthetic prior to catheter placement the patient

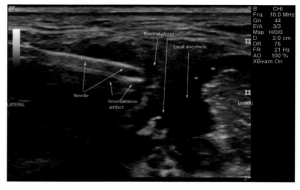

Figure 16.6 Local anesthetic injected through a Tuohy needle: notice the separation of the brachial plexus.

will get the benefit of the block, even if they do not get the benefit of the catheter due to incorrect placement of the catheter.

- Due to the differences in acoustic impedance of local anesthetics and surrounding tissue, a pocket of local anesthetic will make visualization of the needle tip and catheter easier.

Additional considerations

A negative aspiration does not rule out an intravascular injection.

Remain alert to the possibility of intravascular injection if the spread of local anesthetic is not seen, as this may indicate that the local anesthetic is being deposited into a vessel and not perineurally, regardless of a prior negative aspiration.

Whatever total volume of local anesthetic is chosen to be injected, inject all but 10 ml through the needle, saving the last 10 ml to be injected through the catheter itself.

Catheter insertion

Once the catheter is inserted through the Tuohy needle, it will encounter resistance as it exits the tip of the needle. The Tuohy needle must be held in place to facilitate passage of the catheter past its tip. If the needle is not held in place as the catheter is advanced past the tip, pushing the catheter past the initial resistance at the tip of the needle may cause the needle to move deeper. Too much movement of the needle may cause the catheter to be placed in the wrong position.

The goal for catheter insertion is to insert and advance the catheter under direct ultrasound visualization. To accomplish this, the probe must be properly positioned on the patient as the catheter is advanced towards the brachial plexus. Initially, this may be the most difficult part of placing perineural catheters.

There are two ways to accomplish advancing the catheter under direct visualization by an unassisted anesthesiologist.

1. Once the initial injection of local anesthetic is completed, the ultrasound probe is laid on the sterile drape and the extension tubing is gently disconnected from the Tuohy needle. Next, grasp the Tuohy needle and advance the catheter just past the tip of the needle (Figure 16.7). As the catheter is advanced, some resistance may be felt as the catheter exits the tip of the needle. Do not advance the catheter if there is too much

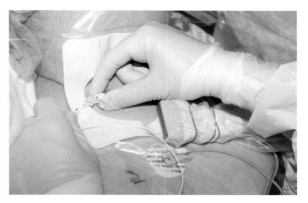

Figure 16.7 With the ultrasound probe on the sterile drape, the Tuohy needle is grasped with one hand while the other hand advances the catheter just past the tip of the needle.

resistance. If this occurs, rotate the tip of the Tuohy needle or pull the needle back 1 to 2 millimeters and try to advance the catheter again. If these maneuvers fail, gently remove the catheter and inject a few milliliters of local anesthetic through the needle under ultrasound visualization to further expand the tissue, then reinsert the catheter into the needle. Once the catheter has passed the tip of the needle, place the probe back on the patient and find the tip of the catheter, which should only be a centimeter or two past the tip of the needle. With the catheter tip past the tip of the needle, the catheter can be advanced under direct ultrasound visualization without having to hold the needle (Figure 16.10).

2. A more advanced method requires the ultrasound probe and Tuohy needle to be held in one hand while advancing the catheter with the other hand. Hold the ultrasound probe between the first and second fingers while holding the needle with the first finger and thumb of the same hand (Figure 16.8). Alternatively, place the thumb from the probe hand beneath the wing of the Tuohy needle to prevent the needle from moving deeper as the catheter is inserted through the needle (Figure 16.9). With the probe and needle stabilized with one hand, the other hand is now free to remove the tubing from the needle and advance the catheter through the needle under direct ultrasound visualization (Figure 16.10).

It is important to watch the catheter as it is advanced. The optimal distance a catheter is inserted

147

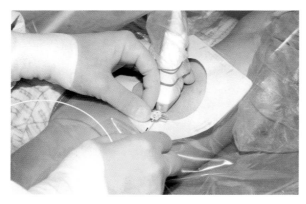

Figure 16.8 The probe is held between the first and second fingers, while the wing of the Tuohy needle is held by the first finger and the thumb.

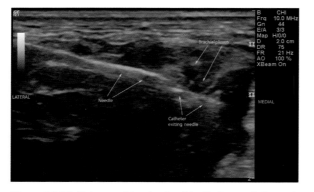

Figure 16.10 Catheter exiting the tip of the Tuohy needle beneath the brachial plexus and in a pocket of local anesthetic.

depends on how the catheter behaves during insertion. As the catheter is advanced, it may either travel straight away from the brachial plexus, without coiling, and poke through the fascial plane containing the local anesthetic from the initial injection or, more likely, begin to coil near the tip of the needle within the space created by the initial local anesthetic bolus. Since the needle tip is near the brachial plexus, the catheter should coil near the brachial plexus, within the correct fascial plane. This is the ideal position for the perineural catheter. When the catheter begins to coil, the entire catheter will not be within the ultrasound beam. Therefore a coiled catheter may only be seen as hyperechoic fragments since only the parts of the coil that cross the ultrasound beam will be visualized. An additional visual confirmation of catheter coiling is movement of tissue within the target fascial plane. Advancing the catheter too

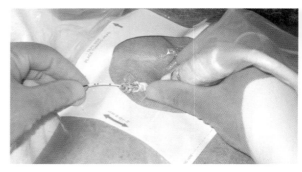

Figure 16.9 The thumb is placed under the wing of the Tuohy needle to prevent movement of the needle as the catheter is inserted.

far may cause excessive coiling of the catheter, and could potentially lead to knotting of the catheter or entrapment of a nerve. Typically, passing the catheter a distance of 3 to 5 cm past the tip of the needle is sufficient.

Additional considerations

Although coiling of the perineural catheter is ideal, it is not mandatory. Allowing the catheter to coil helps protect against migration away from the target structures.

If the perineural catheter advances straight through the fascial plane without coiling, it may be pulled back, under direct ultrasound visualization, into an acceptable position close to the brachial plexus after the Tuohy needle has been removed.

Do not pull the catheter back through the needle as this may cause the catheter to shear on the sharp and angled tip of the Tuohy needle. A sheared catheter may break during reinsertion or during removal by the patient.

Confirmation of catheter position

Once the perineural catheter has been placed in the desired location, hold the catheter in place and slowly back the needle out of the patient over the catheter (Figure 16.11). When the needle is removed, attach a 10-ml syringe of local anesthetic to the catheter. Place the ultrasound probe back on the patient and attempt to find the location of the catheter. Follow the catheter from its skin insertion site through the soft tissue to the brachial plexus or look for hyperechoic lines near the brachial plexus (Figure 16.12). The 19-gage catheter can be difficult to find after it has been inserted. Although the

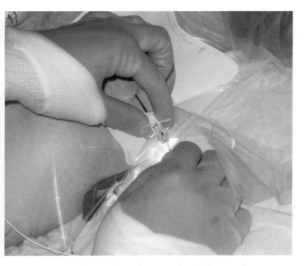

Figure 16.11 Stabilize the catheter as the Tuohy needle is slowly backed out of the patient.

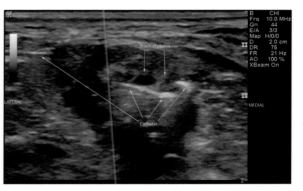

Figure 16.12 Needle is removed and the catheter is positioned beneath the brachial plexus. The tip of the catheter is starting to wrap around the brachial plexus, therefore catheter advancement was stopped. The catheter can be followed from the skin insertion site in the upper left-hand corner of the screen or by looking for hyperechoic areas near the brachial plexus.

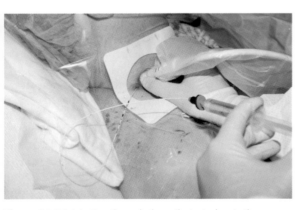

Figure 16.13 Injection through the catheter to locate the catheter tip.

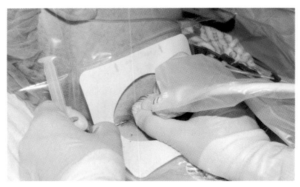

Figure 16.14 Gently pull back on the catheter under ultrasound visualization if the tip has traveled too far from the brachial plexus.

catheter is larger than the 22-gage needles used for the single-injection technique, it does not always travel in a straight path and therefore only a small portion of it will be within the narrow beam of the ultrasound. It may not be possible to know where the *tip* of a coiled catheter is located by scanning alone. Hydrolocation, the injection of small amounts of local anesthetic (or saline) with the accompanying hypoechoic expansion, can aid in locating the *tip* of the catheter. The general location of the catheter should be found first by focused scanning prior to using hydrolocation to find the exact location of the *tip* of the catheter (Figure 16.13). If hydrolocation is the sole technique used to find the catheter itself you may run out of local anesthetic (or saline) before the tip is located. If the tip of the catheter has traveled too far from the brachial plexus, gently pull back on the catheter under direct ultrasound visualization (Figure 16.14). At times it may be necessary to remove the catheter completely and restart the procedure if the optimal position is not obtained, or the catheter position fails to be identified.

Prior to securing the catheter, a 5-ml test dose containing epinephrine is given through the catheter and serves as an additional confirmation that the tip of the catheter is not intravascular.

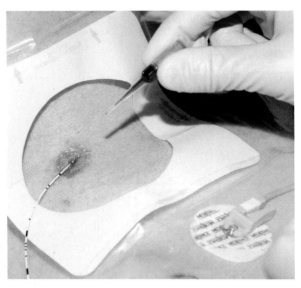

Figure 16.15 Application of a strong skin adhesive to the catheter insertion site: this helps secure the catheter in place and seal the hole made by the large Tuohy needle, preventing leakage of local anesthetic.

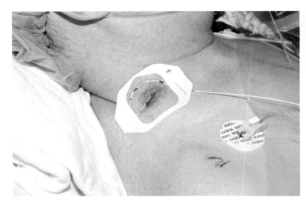

Figure 16.16 Catheter site is dressed with a less strong skin adhesive and a small, clear adhesive dressing.

Additional considerations

Rhythmic pulsation on the syringe plunger (hydro-pulsation) attached to the catheter may cause the tip of the catheter to flicker and move. This may aid in locating the tip of the catheter without using much local anesthetic.

Avoid injecting a large amount of local anesthetic at one time through the catheter without knowing the location of the catheter tip.

A 19-gage catheter, placed through a 17-gage needle, will show injection at the catheter tip much better than a 20-gage catheter.

Avoid using air or an air/liquid mixture to locate the tip of the catheter. Injection of air into the vertebral or carotid arteries can be catastrophic for the patient.

Securing and dressing the catheter site

Once the catheter tip is in the proper location and a negative test dose is confirmed, the catheter may be secured at the skin.

Carefully remove any ultrasound gel from the patient's skin with sterile gauze. A strong skin adhesive or skin glue, such as Dermabond® (Ethicon, Inc.,

Summerville, NJ, USA) or Histoacryl® (B/BRAUN, Germany; TissueSeal, LLC, Ann Arbor, MI, USA) is applied to the catheter insertion site and allowed to dry (Figure 16.15). The adhesive should cover an area approximately 1 to 2 cm around the catheter. The purpose of the skin glue is to seal the catheter insertion site, minimizing catheter movement and leakage of local anesthetic during pump infusion, especially when a patient-controlled analgesia (PCA) function is used.

A wider area around the catheter insertion site is then painted with a less strong liquid adhesive, such as benzoin (Aplicare, Inc., Branford, CT, USA) or Mastisol® (Ferndale Laboratories, Inc., Ferndale, MI, USA) for dressing application. The tail end of the catheter is coiled (to shorten the amount of catheter slack) before placing a transparent adhesive dressing over the entire site (Figure 16.16). The clear dressing allows the patient to monitor for potential signs of infection (e.g., erythema, drainage, or discharge, etc.). After dressing, the catheter is further secured by snapping the injection port into a StatLock® (C.R. Bard, Inc., Covington, GA, USA), which is placed on the patient adjacent to the catheter site.

Additional considerations

Skin glue placed over the catheter insertion site is a key step to prevent leakage of anesthetic and movement of the catheter after it is secured. The less strong adhesives, such as benzoin or Mastisol®, do not form enough of a seal at the catheter insertion site to properly secure the catheter or avoid leaking local anesthetic around the catheter.

Authors' clinical practice

- *Infusion regimen:* for shoulder surgery we use ropivacaine 0.2% at 8 ml/hr with a PCA function of 2 to 5 ml every 30 to 60 minutes. The exact infusion regimen is dependent on the type and extent of surgery, the patient, the patient's history and relevant comorbid conditions, as well as the final location of the catheter in relation to the brachial plexus.
- Although sepsis or untreated bacteremia is considered a relative contraindication for placing a single-injection nerve block, we consider it to be an absolute contraindication for placing a perineural catheter.
- If at any point during the placement of a perineural catheter a vascular puncture occurs, or if blood is aspirated through the catheter, we abort the procedure due to:
  - risk of infection with an indwelling catheter left in a confined space with a surrounding hematoma;
  - potential for increased systemic absorption of local anesthetic being continuously infused under pressure though a damaged vessel wall.
- We do not place continuous catheters in patients who have cervical hardware from previous surgery in order to avoid any risk of an infection compromising the cervical hardware.

Suggested reading

Ilfeld B M, Morey T E, Wright T W, *et al.* (2003). Continuous interscalene brachial plexus block for postoperative pain control at home: a randomized, double-blinded, placebo-controlled study. *Anesth Analg,* **96**(4):1089–95.

Macaire P, Gaertner E, Capdevila X. (2001). Continuous post-operative regional anesthesia at home. *Minerva Anestesiol,* **67**(9 Suppl 1):109–16.

Chapter 7

Supraclavicular continuous perineural catheter

Introduction

Continuous supraclavicular catheters can be used to prolong the duration of analgesia beyond that of a single-injection technique. Continuous catheter placement is considered an advanced technique and it is assumed that the physician has mastered the single-injection supraclavicular technique; therefore a detailed discussion on how to perform a supraclavicular nerve block is not included in this chapter.

Ultrasound anatomy review

Orienting structure: subclavian artery (Figure 17.1)

Equipment

- Ultrasound machine
- High-frequency linear ultrasound probe
- Mayo stand or bedside table
- Sterile gown, sterile gloves, hat, and mask
- Sterile skin preparation
- Sterile drape for the procedure site
- Sterile ultrasound machine controls cover (preferably clear)
- Sterile ultrasound probe sheath with two rubber bands
- Sterile ultrasound conduction gel
- Local anesthetic for skin and subcutaneous infiltration at block needle insertion site
- Blunt-tipped, large-gaged, 4-cm Tuohy needle (17-g needle needed to place 19-g catheter; 18-g needle needed to place 20-g catheter)
- Local anesthetic in 10-ml and 20-ml syringes
- Intravascular test dose containing epinephrine
- Sterile, *flexible* catheter with depth markers
- Catheter adapter for syringe/infusion tubing
- Strong skin adhesive (Dermabond® or Histoacryl®) for securing catheter at insertion site
- Less strong adhesive (benzoin or Mastisol®) for securing clear dressing

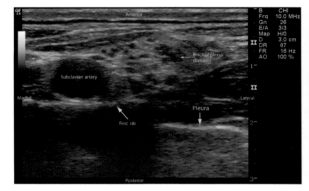

Figure 17.1 Ultrasound view of the left supraclavicular fossa.

Structures that are required to be identified	Structures that may be seen
Subclavian artery	Anterior scalene muscle[1]
First rib	Middle scalene muscle[1]
Divisions of the brachial plexus	Subclavian vein
	Bayonet artifact
	Mirror artifact
	Pleura

Note: [1]May be seen during a confirmatory caudal to cephalad scan.

- *Clear* Tegaderm™ or OpSite™ dressing
- StatLock®
- Illustrated in Figure 17.2

Technique

Technique summary

1. Monitors placed and patient is appropriately sedated
2. Sterile preparation and drape to procedural site

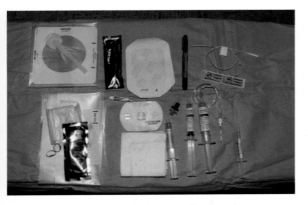

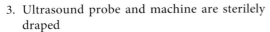

Figure 17.2 Ultrasound-guided perineural catheter kit contents.

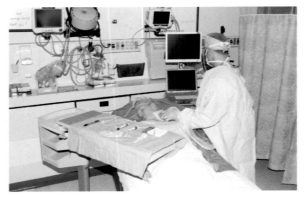

Figure 17.3 Proper set up for the placement of a supraclavicular perineural catheter by an unassisted anesthesiologist.

3. Ultrasound probe and machine are sterilely draped
4. Perform systematic ultrasound scan to find optimal location for catheter insertion
5. Skin wheal is raised
6. Insert Tuohy needle and inject 20 ml of local anesthetic
7. Disconnect tubing from Tuohy needle
8. Insert catheter through Tuohy needle
9. Remove Tuohy needle while catheter held in place
10. Locate catheter on ultrasound image, then incrementally inject 10 ml of local anesthetic through catheter
11. Pull back on catheter as needed to optimize its position
12. Inject test dose containing epinephrine through catheter
13. Catheter insertion site is sealed with strong skin adhesive
14. Catheter is coiled and covered with bezoin and a Tegaderm™
15. Catheter hub is secured to the patient with a StatLock®

Patient and equipment preparation

Since continuous catheters require more time to place than single-injection nerve blocks, require the use of larger gage needles, and the patient's face is often covered with a sterile drape, this procedure may be more uncomfortable and anxiety-provoking for the patient. Use of adequate sedation and an assistant, when possible, to monitor the patient and ensure that

the patient does not reach into the procedural area and contaminate the field may be beneficial.

Continuous perineural catheters should be placed under strict sterile technique with the physician and his/her assistant, when available, wearing a surgical cap, mask, sterile gown, and sterile gloves, as well as sterile covering of the ultrasound transducer and controls. When an assistant is not available, continuous perineural catheters can be placed by an unassisted anesthesiologist (Figure 17.3). The steps taken to prepare the ultrasound machine, probe and catheter kit by an unassisted anesthesiologist are as follows.

1. Position the patient and place the ultrasound machine at the head of the patient's bed, as in the single-injection technique, then drape the ultrasound probe over the front of the ultrasound machine, hanging freely (see Figure 15.3).
2. A block table with the equipment for placing a catheter, sterilely laid out on it, is placed across the patient from the opposite side on which the block is being performed (Figure 17.3).
3. The anesthesiologist should now don the cap, mask, sterile gown, and gloves.
4. Apply a wide sterile preparation to the neck and supraclavicular regions, then place a clear, sterile drape over the area.
5. Conduction gel is then placed inside of the sterile ultrasound probe sheath and the sheath is carefully placed over the hanging probe, then extended over the cord (see Figure 15.4). It is important that the gel is distributed evenly across the tip of the probe and to ensure that there are no air bubbles between the probe and the sheath. A rubber band is then placed across the top of the

153

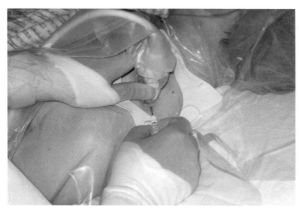

Figure 17.4 Needle inserted in the plane from a lateral to medial direction.

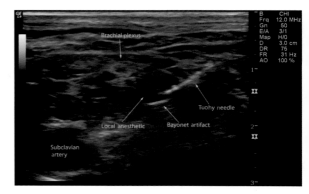

Figure 17.5 Needle is positioned beneath the brachial plexus divisions and local anesthetic injection is carried out.

probe to maintain a snug fit. A second rubber band is then applied lower on the probe to ensure that the sheath does not slide while the probe is being handled (see Figure 15.5).

6. With the probe now covered, the ultrasound machine controls are draped with a clear, sterile cover (see Figure 15.6).

7. A small amount of the remaining sterile conduction gel is placed on the patient, so that scanning can now begin.

Additional considerations

Excessive amounts of ultrasound gel on the patient can make needle and catheter handling very difficult. Only use a minimal amount of conduction gel on the patient.

Scanning

Scanning for perineural catheters is carried out in the same way as for a single-injection supraclavicular brachial plexus block. However, the optimal location for the placement of a catheter may be different than that for a single-injection supracavicular block. Higher concentrations and larger volumes of local anesthetic used in single-injection blocks can overcome a less precise needle placement. Once the effects of the initial bolus have resolved, the infusion of local anesthetic from the catheter tip may not reach all the divisions of the brachial plexus reached by the initial large bolus of local anesthetic, therefore, the placement of the catheter tip needs to be very precise. Scan to find the location where the divisions of the brachial

plexus are the most compact, this may be a few centimeters cephalad to the supraclavicular fossa.

Needle insertion

The Tuohy needle is inserted in plane, as in a single-injection supraclavicular block and advanced under ultrasound visualization towards the brachial plexus in a lateral to medial direction (Figure 17.4). Aim to place the needle, and therefore the catheter, beneath the brachial plexus (Figure 17.5).

Needle insertion should be away from the edge of the probe, not right next to the probe. Inserting the needle away from the probe forces the catheter to travel further before reaching the brachial plexus, as well as forcing the use of a shallow needle-insertion angle. Recall that a shallow needle-insertion angle to the probe will make needle visualization easier. Due to their larger diameter, needles used to place catheters may be visualized even with relatively steep needle-insertion angles. However, a shallow needle-insertion angle is still recommended in order to help secure the catheter and better visualize the catheter once the needle is removed.

Due to the superficial location of the brachial plexus in the supraclavicular fossa in most patients, and the lack of a large muscle to anchor the catheter as it passes through to the brachial plexus, especially in thin patients, only a few centimeters of the catheter may be secured in subcutaneous tissue and muscle; this may increase the risk of catheter movement and dislodgement. Using a shallow insertion angle forces the needle, and therefore the catheter, to travel a greater distance in tissue before reaching your target, which may help stabilize the catheter.

Insertion of a perineural catheter requires the use of a large-bore needle, relative to the needle used for placement of a single-injection block. The number of needle passes made should be kept to a minimum, as these large, blunt needles are capable of considerable tissue trauma. Multiple passes may lead to bruising, pain, and tears of arteries and veins. These large blunt needles can also create channels that allow leakage of local anesthetic after catheter placement. If multiple needle passes are needed, the needle tip should be kept under the skin as the needle is redirected. Multiple skin punctures may increase the probability of local anesthetic leakage, which is problematic for several reasons, as follows.

- Local anesthetic leakage away from the brachial plexus decreases the volume of local anesthetic around the brachial plexus and may lead to catheter failure.
- Wetness from leaking local anesthetic may undo the dressing placed over the catheter insertion site, which may increase the likelihood of catheter dislodgement.
- Wetness at the dressing and dripping of local anesthetic is very uncomfortable for patients and leads to patient requests for early discontinuation of the catheter.

Additional considerations

The most important part of the needle to keep in constant visualization is the needle tip. If the tip is not constantly visualized, one is never certain as to where it is located and what structures it may be penetrating. The only part of the needle that can be visualized is the part that is traveling through the narrow ultrasound beam.

Confusion about the true location of the tip of the needle may cause the needle to be inadvertently advanced into the lung, subclavian artery, or the brachial plexus.

Larger needles used to place continuous catheters may exhibit a bayonet artifact.

Local anesthetic injection and needle repositioning

With the Tuohy needle positioned beneath the brachial plexus, injection of local anesthetic can be carried out. Observe the pattern of spread to confirm positioning of the needle tip within the correct fascial plane. The needle can be repositioned if spread of local anesthetic is not within the correct fascial plane. Injection through the Tuohy needle prior to placement of the catheter serves several purposes, as follows.

- Injection of local anesthetic and observance of the spread, serves as a confirmation as to the location of the needle tip within the correct fascial plane so that the catheter will also be in the correct fascial plane.
- Local anesthetic injection can expand the surrounding tissue and make passage of the catheter easier.
- If the catheter is not positioned in the proper location initially, by injecting some local anesthetic prior to catheter placement the patient will get the benefit of the block, even if they do not get the benefit of the catheter due to incorrect placement of the catheter.
- Due to the differences in acoustic impedance of local anesthetics and surrounding tissue, a pocket of local anesthetic will make visualization of the needle tip and catheter easier.

Additional considerations

A negative aspiration does not rule out an intravascular injection.

Remain alert to the possibility of intravascular injection if the spread of local anesthetic is not seen, as this may indicate that the local anesthetic is being deposited into a vessel and not perineurally, regardless of a prior negative aspiration.

Whatever total volume of local anesthetic is chosen to be injected, inject all but 10 ml through the needle, saving the last 10 ml to be injected through the catheter itself.

Catheter insertion

Once the catheter is inserted through the Tuohy needle, it will encounter resistance as it exits the tip of the needle. The Tuohy needle must be held in place to facilitate passage of the catheter past its tip. If the needle is not held in place as the catheter is advanced past the tip, pushing the catheter past the initial resistance at the tip of the needle may cause the needle to move deeper. Too much movement of the needle may cause the catheter to be placed in the wrong position.

The goal for catheter insertion is to insert and advance the catheter under direct ultrasound visualization. To accomplish this, the probe must be

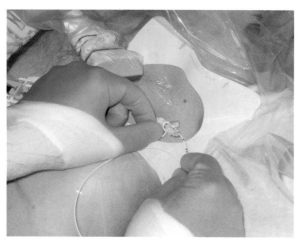

Figure 17.6 With the ultrasound probe on the sterile drape, the Tuohy needle is grasped with one hand while the other hand advances the catheter just past the tip of the needle.

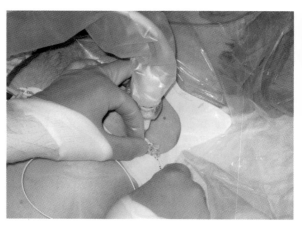

Figure 17.7 The probe is held between the first and second fingers, while the wing of the Tuohy needle is held by the first finger and the thumb.

properly positioned on the patient as the catheter is advanced towards the brachial plexus. Initially, this may be the most difficult part of placing perineural catheters.

There are two ways to accomplish advancing the catheter under direct visualization by an unassisted anesthesiologist.

1. Once the initial injection of local anesthetic is completed, the ultrasound probe is laid on the sterile drape and the extension tubing is gently disconnected from the Tuohy needle. Next, grasp the Tuohy needle and advance the catheter just past the tip of the needle (Figure 17.6). As the catheter is advanced, some resistance may be felt as the catheter exits the tip of the needle. Do not advance the catheter if there is too much resistance. If this occurs, rotate the tip of the Tuohy needle or pull the needle back 1 to 2 millimeters and try to advance the catheter again. If these maneuvers fail, gently remove the catheter and inject a few milliliters of local anesthetic through the needle under ultrasound visualization to further expand the tissue, then reinsert the catheter into the needle. Once the catheter has passed the tip of the needle, place the probe back on the patient and find the tip of the catheter, which should only be a centimeter or two past the tip of the needle. With the catheter tip past the tip of the needle, the catheter can be advanced without having to hold the needle (Figure 17.9).

2. A more advanced method requires the ultrasound probe and Tuohy needle to be held in one hand while advancing the catheter with the other hand. Hold the ultrasound probe between the first and second fingers while holding the needle with the first finger and thumb of the same hand (Figure 17.7). Alternatively, place the thumb from the probe hand beneath the wing of the Tuohy to prevent the needle from moving deeper as the catheter is inserted through the needle (Figure 17.8). With the probe and needle stabilized with one hand, the other hand is now free to remove the tubing from the needle and advance the catheter through the needle under direct ultrasound visualization (Figure 17.9). Deeper movement of the needle may cause the catheter to be placed in the wrong position, a vascular puncture or a pneumothorax.

It is important to watch the catheter as it is advanced. The optimal distance a catheter is inserted depends on how the catheter behaves during insertion. As the catheter is advanced, it may either travel straight away from the brachial plexus, without coiling, and poke through the fascial plane containing the local anesthetic from the initial injection or, more likely, begin to coil near the tip of the needle within the space created by the initial local anesthetic bolus. Since the needle tip is near the brachial plexus, the catheter should coil near the brachial plexus,

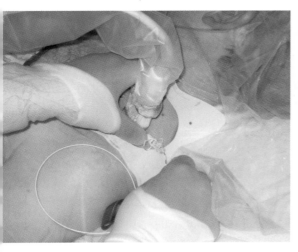

Figure 17.8 The thumb is placed under the wing of the Tuohy needle to prevent movement of the needle as the catheter is inserted.

within the correct fascial plane. This is the ideal position for the perineural catheter. When the catheter begins to coil, the entire catheter will not be within the ultrasound beam. Therefore a coiled catheter may only be seen as hyperechoic fragments since only the parts of the coil that cross the ultrasound beam will be visualized. An additional visual confirmation of catheter coiling is movement of tissue within the target fascial plane. Advancing the catheter too far may cause excessive coiling of the catheter, and could potentially lead to knotting of the catheter or entrapment of a nerve. Typically, passing the catheter a distance of 3 to 5 cm past the tip of the needle is sufficient.

Additional considerations

Although coiling of the perineural catheter is ideal, it is not mandatory. Allowing the catheter to coil helps protect against migration away from the target structures.

If the perineural catheter advances straight through the fascial plane without coiling, it may be pulled back, under direct ultrasound visualization, into an acceptable position close to the brachial plexus after the Tuohy needle has been removed.

Do not pull the catheter back through the needle as this may cause the catheter to shear on the sharp and angled tip of the Tuohy needle. A sheared catheter may break during reinsertion or during removal by the patient.

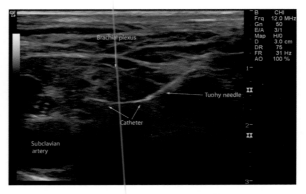

Figure 17.9 Catheter is exiting the needle and has not started to coil.

Confirmation of catheter position

Once the perineural catheter has been placed in the desired location beneath the brachial plexus, hold the catheter in place and slowly back the needle out of the patient over the catheter (Figure 17.10). When the needle is removed, attach a 10-ml syringe of local anesthetic to the catheter. Place the ultrasound probe back on the patient and attempt to find the location of the catheter. Follow the catheter from its skin insertion site through the soft tissue to the brachial plexus or look for hyperechoic lines near the brachial plexus (Figure 17.11). The 19-gage catheter can be difficult to find after it has been inserted. Although the catheter is larger than the 22-gage needles used for the single-injection technique, it does not always travel in a straight path and therefore only a small portion of it will be within the narrow beam of the ultrasound. It may not be possible to know where the *tip* of a coiled catheter is located by scanning alone. Hydrolocation, the injection of small amounts of local anesthetic (or saline) with the accompanying hypoechoic expansion, can aid in locating the *tip* of the catheter. The general location of the catheter should be found first by focused scanning prior to using hydrolocation to find the exact location of the *tip* of the catheter. If hydrolocation is the sole technique used to find the catheter itself you may run out of local anesthetic (or saline) before the tip is located. If the tip of the catheter has traveled too far from the brachial plexus, gently pull back on the catheter under direct ultrasound visualization. At times it may be necessary to remove the catheter completely and restart the procedure if the optimal position is not obtained, or the catheter position fails to be identified.

157

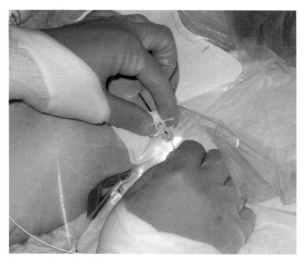

Figure 17.10 Stabilize the catheter as the Tuohy needle is slowly backed out of the patient.

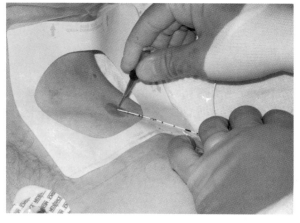

Figure 17.12 Application of a strong skin adhesive to the catheter insertion site. This helps secure the catheter in place and seal the hole made by the large Tuohy needle, preventing leakage of local anesthetic.

Prior to securing the catheter, a 5-ml test dose containing epinephrine is given through the catheter and serves as an additional confirmation that the tip of the catheter is not intravascular.

Additional considerations

Rhythmic pulsation on the syringe plunger (hydro-pulsation) attached to the catheter may cause the tip of the catheter to flicker. This may aid in locating the tip of the catheter without using much local anesthetic.

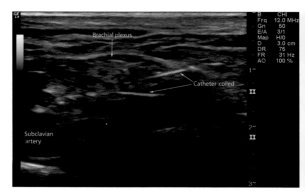

Figure 17.11 Needle has been removed and the catheter is coiled beneath the brachial plexus. The catheter can be followed from the skin insertion site to the brachial plexus.

Avoid injecting a large amount of local anesthetic at one time through the catheter without knowing the location of the catheter tip.

A 19-gage catheter, placed through a 17-gage needle, will show injection at the catheter tip much better than a 20-gage catheter.

Avoid using air or an air/liquid mixture to locate the tip of the catheter for blocks above the clavicle.

Securing and dressing the catheter site

Once the catheter tip is in the proper location and a negative test dose is confirmed, the catheter may be secured at the skin.

Carefully remove any ultrasound gel from the patient's skin with sterile gauze. A strong skin adhesive or skin glue, such as Dermabond® (Ethicon, Inc., Summerville, NJ, USA) or Histoacryl® (B/BRAUN, Germany; TissueSeal, LLC, Ann Arbor, MI, USA) is applied to the catheter insertion site and allowed to dry (Figure 17.12). The adhesive should cover an area approximately 1 to 2 cm around the catheter. The purpose of the skin glue is to seal the catheter insertion site, minimizing catheter movement and leakage of local anesthetic during pump infusion, especially when a patient-controlled analgesia (PCA) function is used.

A wider area around the catheter insertion site is then painted with a less strong liquid adhesive, such as benzoin (Aplicare, Inc., Branford, CT, USA) or Mastisol® (Ferndale Laboratories, Inc., Ferndale, MI, USA) for dressing application. The tail end of the

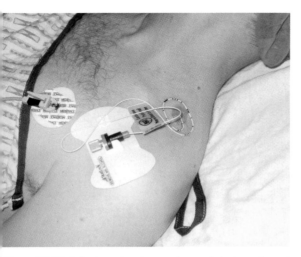

Figure 17.13 Fully dressed and secured supraclavicular perineural catheter with StatLock®.

catheter is coiled (to shorten the amount of catheter slack) before placing a transparent adhesive dressing over the entire site. The clear dressing allows the patient to monitor for potential signs of infection (e.g., erythema, drainage, or discharge, etc.). After dressing, the catheter is further secured by snapping the injection port into a StatLock® (C. R. Bard, Inc., Covington, GA, USA), which is placed on the patient adjacent to the catheter site (Figure 17.13).

Additional considerations

Skin glue placed over the catheter insertion site is a key step to prevent leakage of anesthetic and movement of the catheter after it is secured. The less strong adhesives, such as benzoin or Mastisol®, do not form enough of a seal at the catheter insertion site to properly secure the catheter or avoid leaking local anesthetic around the catheter.

Authors' clinical practice

- *Infusion regimen*: for shoulder surgery we use ropivacaine 0.2% at 8 ml/hr with a PCA function of 2 to 5 ml every 30 to 60 minutes. The exact infusion regimen is dependent on the type and

extent of surgery, the patient, the patient's history and relevant comorbid conditions, as well as the final location of the catheter in relation to the brachial plexus.

- *Infusion regimen*: for surgery on the arm, forearm, or hand, we use ropivacaine 0.2% or ropivacaine 0.3% at 10 ml/hr with a PCA function of 2 to 5 ml every 30 to 60 minutes. The exact infusion regimen is dependent on the type and extent of surgery, the patient, the patient's history and relevant comorbid conditions, as well as the final location of the catheter in relation to the brachial plexus.

- Although sepsis or untreated bacteremia is considered a relative contraindication for placing a single-injection nerve block, we consider it to be an absolute contraindication for placing a perineural catheter.

- If at any point during the placement of a perineural catheter a vascular puncture occurs, or if blood is aspirated through the catheter, we abort the procedure due to:
  - risk of infection with an indwelling catheter left in a confined space with a surrounding hematoma;
  - potential for increased systemic absorption of local anesthetic being continuously infused under pressure though a damaged vessel wall.

- We do not place continuous catheters in patients who have cervical hardware from previous surgery in order to avoid any risk of an infection compromising the cervical hardware.

Suggested reading

Ilfeld B M, Morey T E, Wright T W, *et al.* (2003). Continuous interscalene brachial plexus block for postoperative pain control at home: a randomized, double-blinded, placebo-controlled study. *Anesth Analg*, **96**(4):1089–95.

Macaire P, Gaertner E, Capdevila X. (2001). Continuous post-operative regional anesthesia at home. *Minerva Anestesiol*, **67**(9 Suppl 1):109–16.

18 Infraclavicular continuous perineural catheter

Introduction

When the ultrasound single-injection infraclavicular brachial plexus block technique is advanced to a perineural catheter technique, it is able to provide a longer duration of postoperative analgesia for several upper extremity procedures. This approach works best when providing analgesia for distal upper extremity procedures, primarily for any procedure below the elbow. Like the non-catheter technique, the placement of an infraclavicular perineural catheter is performed at the anterior shoulder and chest wall, in the area of the deltopectoral groove. Here, the perineural catheter can be positioned next to the cords of the brachial plexus as they travel distally towards the axilla. Although placement of an ultrasound-guided brachial plexus perineural catheter and an ultrasound-guided non-catheter brachial plexus block are similar, advancement to placing a catheter should not occur until proficiency has been achieved with the single-injection technique.

Ultrasound anatomy review

Orienting structure: axillary artery (Figure 18.1)

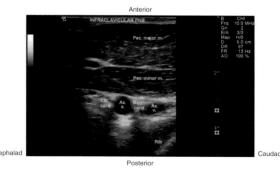

Figure 18.1 Normal infraclavicular ultrasound anatomy at the deltopectoral groove.

Structures that are required to be identified	Structures that may be seen
Axillary artery	Pectoralis major muscle
Axillary vein	Pectoralis minor muscle
Cords of brachial plexus	Rib/lung
	Anomalous vasculature

Equipment

- Ultrasound machine
- High-frequency ultrasound probe
- Mayo stand or bedside table
- Sterile gown, sterile gloves, hat, and mask
- Sterile skin preparation
- Sterile drape for the procedure site
- Sterile ultrasound controls cover (preferably clear)
- Sterile ultrasound probe sheath with two rubber bands
- Sterile ultrasound gel
- Local anesthetic for skin and subcutaneous infiltration at block needle insertion site
- Blunt-tipped, large-gaged, 8-cm Tuohy needle (17-gage needle needed to place 19-gage catheter; 18-gage needle needed to place 20-gage catheter)
- Local anesthetic in 10-ml and 20-ml syringes
- Intravascular test dose containing epinephrine
- Sterile, *flexible* catheter with depth markers
- Catheter adapter for syringe/infusion tubing
- Strong skin adhesive, such as Dermabond® (Ethicon, Inc., Summerville, NJ, USA) or Histoacryl® (B/BRAUN, Germany; TissueSeal, LLC, Ann Arbor, MI, USA), for securing catheter at insertion site

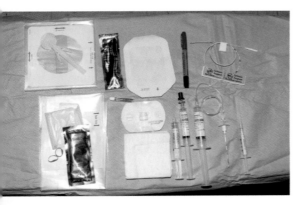

Figure 18.2 Ultrasound-guided perineural catheter kit contents.

- Less strong adhesive, such as benzoin (Aplicare, Inc., Branford, CT, USA) or Mastisol® (Ferndale Laboratories, Inc., Ferndale, MI, USA) for securing clear dressing
- *Clear* Tegaderm™ (3M Health Care, St. Paul, MN, USA) dressing
- StatLock® (Venetec International, San Diego, CA, USA) or similar device
- Illustrated in Figure 18.2

Technique
Technique summary

1. Monitors placed and patient is appropriately sedated
2. Sterile preparation and drape to procedural site
3. Ultrasound probe and machine are sterilely draped
4. Perform systematic ultrasound scan to find optimal location for catheter insertion
5. Skin wheal is raised
6. Insert Tuohy needle and inject 30 ml of local anesthetic
7. Disconnect tubing from Tuohy needle
8. Insert catheter through Tuohy needle
9. Remove Tuohy needle while catheter is held in place
10. Locate catheter on ultrasound image, then incrementally inject 10 ml of local anesthetic through catheter
11. Pull back on catheter as needed to optimize its position
12. Inject test dose containing epinephrine through catheter

13. Catheter insertion site is sealed with strong skin adhesive
14. Catheter is coiled and covered with benzoin and a Tegaderm™
15. Catheter hub is secured to the patient with a StatLock® or similar device

Patient and equipment preparation

Since continuous catheters require more time to place than single-injection nerve blocks, require the use of larger gage needles, and the patient's face is often covered with a sterile drape, this procedure may be more uncomfortable and anxiety provoking for the patient. Use of adequate sedation and an assistant, when possible, to monitor the patient and ensure that the patient does not reach into the procedural area and contaminate the field may be beneficial.

Continuous perineural catheters should be placed under strict sterile technique with the physician and his/her assistant, when available, wearing a surgical cap, mask, sterile gown, and sterile gloves, as well as sterile covering of the ultrasound transducer and controls. When an assistant is not available, continuous perineural catheters can be placed by an unassisted anesthesiologist (Figure 18.3). The steps taken to prepare the ultrasound machine, probe, and catheter kit by an unassisted anesthesiologist are as follows.

1. Position the patient and place the ultrasound machine at the head of the patient's bed, as in the single-injection technique, then drape the ultrasound probe over the front of the ultrasound machine, hanging freely (see Figure 15.3).
2. A block table with the equipment for placing a catheter, sterilely laid out on it, is placed across the patient from the opposite side on which the block will be performed (Figure 18.3).
3. The anesthesiologist should now don the cap, mask, sterile gown, and gloves.
4. Apply a wide sterile preparation to the deltopectoral and supraclavicular regions, then place a clear, sterile drape over the area.
5. Conduction gel is then placed inside the sterile ultrasound probe sheath and the sheath is then carefully placed over the hanging probe, then extended over the cord (see Figure 15.4). It is important that the gel is distributed evenly across

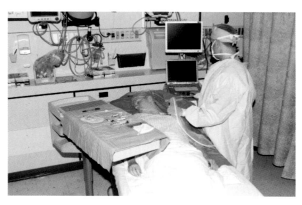

Figure 18.3 Proper set-up for the placement of an infraclavicular perineural catheter by an unassisted anesthesiologist.

the tip of the probe to ensure that there are no air bubbles between the probe and the sheath.

A rubber band is then placed across the top of the probe to maintain a snug fit. A second rubber band is then applied lower on the probe to ensure that the sheath does not slide while the probe is being handled (see Figure 15.5).

6. With the probe now covered, the ultrasound machine controls are draped with a clear, sterile cover (see Figure 15.6).

7. **A** small amount of the remaining sterile conduction gel is placed on the patient, so that scanning can now begin.

Additional considerations

Excessive amounts of conduction gel on the patient can make needle and catheter handling very difficult. Only use a minimal amount of conduction gel on the patient.

Scanning

Scanning for perineural catheters is carried out in the same way as for a single-injection infraclavicular brachial plexus block. However, placement for the catheter tip needs to be more precise than that for a single injection. Higher concentrations and larger volumes of local anesthetic used in single-injection blocks can overcome a less precise needle placement. Once the effects of the initial bolus have resolved, the infusion of the local anesthetic from the catheter tip may not reach all the structures affected by the initial bolus of

local anesthetic unless positioned optimally. Therefore, a systematic scan should be performed to find an ideal position in the infraclavicular region to place the perineural catheter. Here the target structures should be positioned away from the lung, no anomalous vasculature should be in the vicinity of the posterior cord, and the tissue cephalad to the target structures should be free of any significant vascular structures so that the posterior cord is easily accessible by a large-bore needle.

Needle insertion

The needle is inserted and guided *in plane* with the ultrasound beam, just as in a single-injection infraclavicular block. The needle should travel in a cephalad to caudad direction, posteriorly towards the cords of the brachial plexus (Figure 18.4a and b). Make certain to visualize the needle and always be aware of where the needle tip is throughout the procedure. The path of the needle should be aimed just posterior to the axillary artery. The needle positioning for placement of a perineural catheter is different than when placing a single-injection infraclavicular block. The ideal initial needle tip placement before injection of local anesthetic should be next to the lateral cord, not the posterior cord (Figure 18.5). This will minimize the number of needle passes required for the following steps in the placement of the perineural catheter. Special care should be taken to avoid contacting the cords of the brachial plexus in order to minimize the potential for nerve damage.

Insertion of a perineural catheter requires the use of a large-bore needle, relative to the needle used for placement of a single-injection block. Due to their larger diameter, needles used to place catheters may be more easily visualized by the ultrasound, even with relatively steep needle-insertion angles. The larger gage needles, though, also present some potential problems. First, they often cause more discomfort for the patient, so we recommend not only raising a skin wheal with local anesthetic prior to inserting the large needle, but also infiltrating some of the subcutaneous tissue and pectoralis muscle with local anesthetic along the potential path of the large needle. Second, the large, blunt-tipped needles used for placement of the catheters can create channels that allow leakage of local anesthetic after catheter placement. Multiple passes with these large needles will increase the probability of local anesthetic leakage from the

(a)

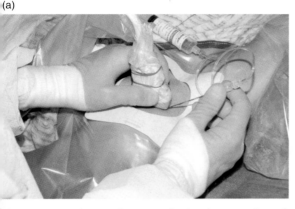

(b)

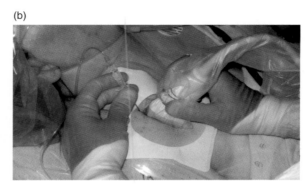

Figure 18.4 In-plane needle position for the placement of an infraclavicular perineural catheter.

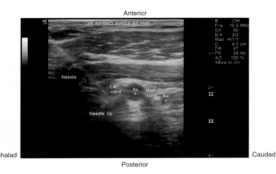

Figure 18.5 Ideal initial needle position for an infraclavicular perineural catheter prior to local anesthetic injection.

targeted area and lead to patient discomfort. If several needle passes are required, do not take the needle out of the skin and create another hole in the skin, but rather redirect the needle in the subcutaneous tissue through the same skin hole already created. Multiple holes in the skin can lead to leaking of local anesthetic and wetness under the dressing, which can loosen the dressing and dislodge the catheter. Also, try to create as few holes as possible in the fascia posterior to the pectoralis minor muscle to minimize the channels for potential leakage of the local anesthetic away from its target structures. Third, large blunt needles can create tears in arteries and veins, which can lead to bleeding and hematomas.

Additional considerations

The most important part of the needle to keep in constant visualization is the needle tip. If the tip is not constantly visualized, one is never certain as to where it is located and what structures it may be penetrating. The only part of the needle that can be visualized is the part that is traveling through the narrow ultrasound beam.

Do not touch the brachial plexus cords with the Tuohy needle.

Local anesthetic injection and needle repositioning

Injection through the Tuohy needle prior to placement of the perineural catheter serves several purposes, as follows.

- Injection of local anesthetic and visualization of the spread serves as a confirmation that the location of the needle is within the correct fascial plane, so the catheter should also pass within the correct fascial plane.
- Local anesthetic injection can expand the surrounding tissue and make passage of the catheter easier.
- If the catheter ends up positioned incorrectly, the injection of some local anesthetic prior to catheter placement will give the patient, at the very least, the benefit of a single-injection block, even if they do not get the benefit of the catheter due to incorrect placement.
- Due to the differences in acoustic impedance of local anesthetics and the surrounding tissue, a pocket of local anesthetic will make the visualization of the needle tip and perineural catheter easier.

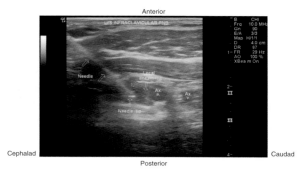

Figure 18.6 Initial injection of local anesthetic at the lateral cord.

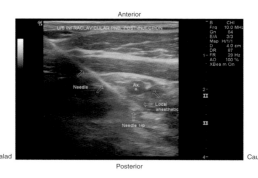

Figure 18.7 Further injection of local anesthetic at the posterior cord.

What makes the initial injection of local anesthetic during the placement of a perineural catheter at the infraclavicular region different from that of a non-catheter technique begins with the site of initial injection. The needle tip should be initially positioned adjacent to the lateral cord, instead of the posterior cord. Once this position is obtained, approximately ¼ to ⅓ of the initial volume of local anesthetic to be injected is deposited. As with the non-catheter blocks, negative aspiration is confirmed before the initial injection, after approximately every 3 to 5 ml of injection, and every time the needle is repositioned. If there is high resistance to injection, stop and reposition the needle. Be certain to visualize expansion of the hypoechoic local anesthetic in its well contained space around the lateral cord, and its spread around the axillary artery toward the posterior and medial cords (Figure 18.6). Appropriate spread of local anesthetic to all three cords will likely not be obtained by injection solely at this site. Once the desired volume of local anesthetic is injected at the lateral cord, the needle is then advanced along its original trajectory toward the posterior cord and the remaining volume of local anesthetic is injected. As always, it is important to visualize the spread of local anesthetic within the well defined space, reaching all three cords (Figure 18.7). The tip of the needle can be advanced slightly past the posterior cord in order to achieve more spread of local anesthetic toward the medial cord, if necessary. After the injection of the full amount of local anesthetic to be deposited through the needle is complete, ensure that the needle tip is positioned near the posterior cord, within the now dilated fascial plane containing the brachial plexus. This will allow for advancement and coiling of the perineural catheter at the posterior cord. Several studies have shown that a single injection of

local anesthetic at the posterior cord yields the highest success rate when performing an infraclavicular brachial plexus block. This is likely because the local anesthetic is able to travel a short distance both cephalad and caudad around the axillary artery to reach the lateral and medial cords, respectively. Therefore, we aim to position the perineural catheter near the posterior cord to run our perineural infusions.

Additional considerations

A negative aspiration does not rule out an intravascular injection.

Remain alert to the possibility of intravascular injection if the spread of local anesthetic is not seen, as this may indicate that the local anesthetic is being deposited into a vessel and not perineurally, regardless of a prior negative aspiration.

Whatever total volume of local anesthetic is chosen to be injected, inject all but 10 ml through the needle, saving the last 10 ml to be injected through the catheter itself.

Catheter insertion

Once the catheter is inserted through the Tuohy needle, it will encounter resistance as it exits the tip of the needle. The Tuohy needle must be held in place to facilitate passage of the catheter past its tip. If the needle is not held in place as the catheter is advanced past the tip, pushing the catheter past the initial resistance at the tip of the needle may cause the needle to move deeper. Too much movement of the needle may cause the catheter to be placed in the wrong position.

The goal for catheter insertion is to insert and advance the catheter under direct ultrasound visualization. To accomplish this, the probe must be properly positioned on the patient as the catheter is advanced towards the brachial plexus. Initially, this may be the most difficult part of placing perineural catheters.

There are two ways to accomplish advancing the catheter under direct visualization by an unassisted anesthesiologist.

1. Once the initial injection of local anesthetic is completed, the ultrasound probe is laid on the sterile drape and the extension tubing is gently disconnected from the Tuohy needle. Next, grasp the Tuohy needle with one hand and advance the catheter just past the tip of the needle with the other hand (Figure 18.8). As the catheter is advanced, some resistance may be felt as the catheter exits the tip of the needle. Do not advance the catheter if there is too much resistance. If this

occurs, rotate the tip of the Tuohy needle or pull the needle back 1 to 2 millimeters and try to advance the catheter again. If these maneuvers fail, gently remove the catheter and inject a few milliliters of local anesthetic through the needle under ultrasound visualization to further expand the tissue, then reinsert the catheter into the needle. Once the catheter has passed the tip of the Tuohy needle, place the probe back on the patient and find the tip of the catheter, which should only be one to two centimeters past the tip of the needle. With the catheter tip past the tip of the Tuohy needle, the catheter can be advanced under direct ultrasound visualization without having to hold the needle.

2. A more advanced method requires holding the ultrasound probe and Tuohy needle in one hand while advancing the catheter with the other hand. When ready to advance the catheter, hold the ultrasound probe in a manner so that some fingers are free to also hold and stabilize the Tuohy needle. There are a few different ways to do this, depending on hand size and comfort of the physician. One way to do this has the physician holding the ultrasound probe firmly in the palm of the hand, between the base of the thumb and first finger, while holding the shaft or hub of the Tuohy needle between the tips of the thumb and first or second finger (Figure 18.9a and b). Another way to do this can have the physician holding the probe between the thumb and first finger, while stabilizing the needle between the first and second fingers (Figure 18.10a and b).

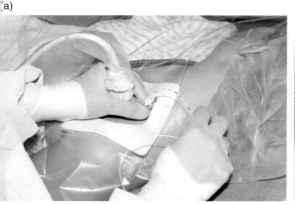

Figure 18.8 With the ultrasound probe lying on the sterile drape, the Tuohy needle is grasped in one hand while the other advances the catheter just past the tip of the Tuohy needle.

(a)

(b)

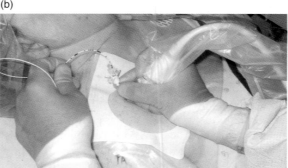

Figure 18.9 Advancement of a perineural catheter through a needle under ultrasound visualization while holding the probe in the palm of the hand and the Tuohy needle between the thumb and first or second finger.

(a)

(b)

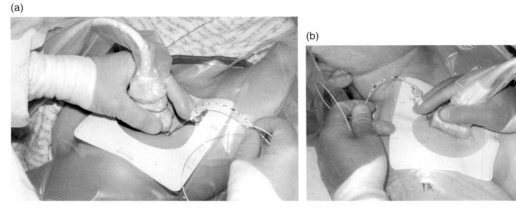

Figure 18.10 Advancement of a perineural catheter through a needle under ultrasound visualization while holding the Tuohy needle between the first and second fingers.

Either way, the key point is to stabilize both the ultrasound probe and the needle with one hand. There is now a free hand to remove the extension tubing from the Tuohy needle and advance the catheter through the needle. The Tuohy needle must be held firmly between the finger tips due to the resistance that is encountered by the catheter as it exits the tip of the needle.

It is important to watch the catheter as it is advanced. The optimal distance a catheter is inserted depends on how it behaves during insertion. As the catheter is advanced, it may either travel straight away from the brachial plexus, without coiling, and poke through the fascial plane containing the local anesthetic from the initial injection or, more likely, begin to coil near the tip of the needle within the space created by the initial local anesthetic bolus. Since the needle tip is near the brachial plexus, the catheter should coil near the brachial plexus, within the correct fascial plane. This is the ideal position for the perineural catheter. When the catheter begins to coil, the entire catheter will not be within the ultrasound beam. Therefore, a coiled catheter may only be seen as hyperechoic fragments since only the parts of the coil that cross the ultrasound beam will be visualized. An additional visual confirmation of catheter coiling is movement of tissue within the target fascial plane. Advancing the catheter too far may cause excessive coiling of the catheter, and could potentially lead to knotting of the catheter or entrapment of a nerve. Typically, passing the catheter a distance of 3 to 5 cm past the tip of the needle is sufficient.

Additional considerations

Although coiling of the perineural catheter is ideal, it is not mandatory. Allowing the catheter to coil helps protect against migration away from the target structures.

If the perineural catheter advances straight through the fascial plane without coiling, it may be pulled back into an acceptable position close to the posterior cord, under ultrasound guidance, after the Tuohy needle has been removed.

Do not pull the catheter back through the needle as this may cause the catheter to shear on the sharp and angled tip of the Tuohy needle. A sheared catheter may break during reinsertion or during removal by the patient.

Confirmation of catheter position

Once the perineural catheter has been placed in the desired location, hold the catheter in place and slowly back the needle out of the patient over the catheter (Figure 18.11). When the needle is removed, attach a 10-ml syringe of local anesthetic to the catheter. Next, place the ultrasound probe back on the patient and attempt to visualize the catheter by either tracing the catheter through the soft issue from its insertion site or by looking for the catheter, seen as hyperechoic lines, near the brachial plexus. The 19-gage catheter can be difficult to find after it has been inserted. Although the catheter is larger than the 21-gage needles used for the single-injection technique, it does not always travel in a straight path and therefore only

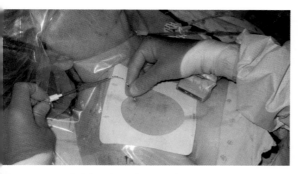

Figure 18.11 Stabilize the catheter and remove the needle from the patient while the catheter remains in place.

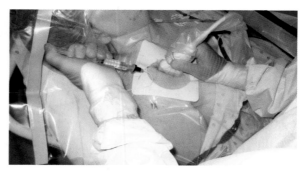

Figure 18.12 Injection through the catheter to locate the catheter tip.

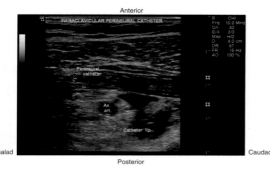

Figure 18.13 Ideal position of an infraclavicular perineural catheter tip near the posterior cord.

a small portion of it will be within the narrow beam of the ultrasound. It is very difficult to identify the tip of the catheter solely by scanning when the catheter is coiled in the fascial plane. The hydrolocation technique can help identify the catheter tip. To do this, first visualize a portion of the catheter near the cords of the brachial plexus then administer very small, pulsing injections of local anesthetic (or saline) through the catheter (Figure 18.12). There will be an accompanying hypoechoic expansion at the tip of the catheter with every small injection of local anesthetic. If the tip of the catheter has been positioned too far from the posterior cord, gently pull back on the catheter, watching it move under direct ultrasound visualization, until the tip is optimally positioned adjacent to the posterior cord (Figure 18.13). Here the remainder of the local anesthetic can be injected, and spread of local anesthetic to all three cords should be observed. At times it may be necessary to remove the catheter completely and restart the procedure if the optimal position is not obtained, or the catheter position fails to be identified.

Just prior to securing the perineural catheter, a test dose containing epinephrine is administered through the catheter to serve as an additional confirmation that the tip of the catheter is not intravascular.

Additional considerations

If the hydrolocation technique is used to find the catheter initially, before a focused scan for the catheter at the brachial plexus is performed, one may run out of local anesthetic before the tip of the catheter can be identified.

Rhythmic pulsation on the syringe plunger (hydropulsation) attached to the catheter may cause the tip of the catheter to flicker. This may aid in locating the tip of the catheter without using much local anesthetic.

Avoid injecting a large amount of local anesthetic at one time through the catheter without knowing the location of the catheter tip.

A 19-gage catheter, placed through a 17-gage needle, will show injection at the catheter tip much better than a 20-gage catheter.

If one is having significant difficulty identifying the location of the catheter and/or its tip, one can inject a small amount of air through the catheter while watching the ultrasound screen. The air should show up as a hyperechoic artifact that originates from the catheter tip.

Securing and dressing the catheter at the skin

Once the catheter tip is in the proper location and a negative test dose is confirmed, the catheter may be secured at the skin.

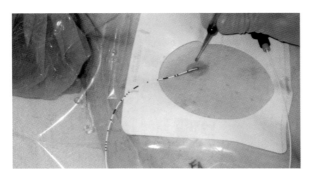

Figure 18.14 Application of a strong skin adhesive to the catheter insertion site. This helps secure the catheter in place and seal the hole made by the large Tuohy needle, preventing leakage of local anesthetic.

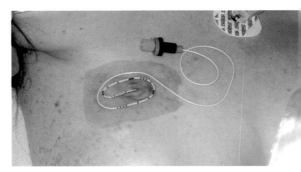

Figure 18.15 Catheter site is dressed with a less strong skin adhesive and a small, clear adhesive dressing.

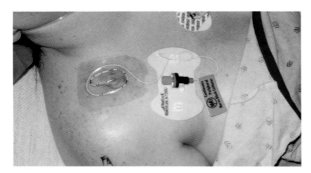

Figure 18.16 Fully dressed and secured infraclavicular perineural catheter with StatLock.®

Carefully remove any ultrasound gel from the patient's skin with sterile gauze. Strong skin adhesive or skin glue, such as Dermabond® (Ethicon, Inc., Summerville, NJ, USA) or Histoacryl® (B/BRAUN, Germany; TissueSeal, LLC, Ann Arbor, MI, USA) is applied to the catheter insertion site and allowed to dry (Figure 18.14). The adhesive should cover an area approximately 1 to 2 cm around the catheter. The purpose of the skin glue is to seal the catheter insertion site, minimizing catheter movement and leakage of local anesthetic during pump infusion, especially when a patient-controlled analgesia (PCA) function is used.

A wider area around the catheter insertion site is then painted with a less strong liquid adhesive, such as benzoin (Aplicare, Inc., Branford, CT, USA) or Mastisol® (Ferndale Laboratories, Inc., Ferndale, MI, USA) for dressing application. The tail end of the catheter is coiled (to shorten the amount of catheter slack) before placing a transparent adhesive dressing over the entire site (Figure 18.15). The clear dressing

allows the patient to monitor for potential signs of infection (e.g., erythema, drainage, discharge, etc.). After dressing, the catheter is further secured by snapping the injection port into a StatLock® (C. R. Bard, Inc., Covington, GA, USA), which is placed on the patient adjacent to the catheter site (Figure 18.16).

Additional considerations

Skin glue placed over the catheter insertion site is a key step to prevent leakage of anesthetic and movement of the catheter after it is secured. The less strong adhesives, such as benzoin or Mastisol®, do not form enough of a seal at the catheter insertion site to properly secure the catheter or avoid leaking local anesthetic around the catheter.

Authors' clinical practice

- *Infusion regimen:* we have found the most success using 0.2% to 0.3% ropivacaine at a higher basal infusion rate of 10 ml/hr plus a PCA of 2 to 5 ml every 30 to 60 minutes. With our current pump volumes of 550 ml, this typically allows the patient to have good analgesia from the perineural catheter for approximately 2 to 2½ days after discharge from the PACU. What determines whether we use 0.2% vs. 0.3% ropivacaine as our infusate is the extent of the procedure for which the catheter is being placed. More extensive and more distal procedures, where there are more nerve endings, are more likely to receive 0.3% ropivacaine as the infusate.
- The total dose of our initial injection for placement of the perineural catheters is the same

as when a single-injection nerve block is performed, except that the last 10 ml are injected through the catheter after it has been positioned.

- Although sepsis or untreated bacteremia is considered a relative contraindication to placing a single-injection nerve block, we consider it to be an absolute contraindication to placing a perineural catheter.
- If a vascular puncture occurs at any point during the placement of a perineural catheter we abort the procedure. Our concerns in this situation include risk for infection with an indwelling catheter left in a confined space with a surrounding hematoma, and potential for intravascular leakage of local anesthetic being continuously infused under pressure.
- When performing the initial sterile preparation at the infraclavicular region, we recommend preparing the supraclavicular region as well. When the structures at the infraclavicular region are located too deeply to be visualized well, or there is anomalous vasculature obstructing the safe performance of the block, one can simply slide the ultrasound probe to the more superficial and consistent anatomy of the supraclavicular region to perform the block without having to stop, reprepare and drape the new site, and change sterile gown and gloves.
- If local anesthetic spread does not reach the medial cord after injection around the posterior and lateral cords, advance the needle just past the posterior cord. One can also torque the needle up underneath the artery toward the medial cord, placing the needle tip around the four- to

five-o'clock position, then re-inject and observe the local anesthetic spread. When placing perineural catheters, we prefer to avoid completely redirecting the Tuohy needle superficial to the axillary artery toward the medial cord, as described in the single-injection technique. This can minimize the needle passes and reduce the risk of vascular puncture (axillary vein) with a large-gage needle. Also, by advancing the needle tip just past the posterior cord to reach the medial cord with local anesthetic, one is able to simply just pull the needle back to the posterior cord before placing the perineural catheter rather than repositioning it entirely, as would be necessary if one approached the medial cord superficial to the axillary artery.

- We have found that it is not necessary to tunnel the perineural catheter to secure it, as long as the steps described in this chapter are performed.

Suggested reading

Ilfeld B M, Le L T, Ramjohn J, *et al.* (2009). The effects of local anesthetic concentration and dose on continuous infraclavicular nerve blocks: a multicenter, randomized, observer-masked, controlled study. *Anesth Analg*, **108**(1):345–50.

Ilfeld B M, Torey T E, Enneking F K. (2004). Infraclavicular perineural local anesthetic infusion: a comparison of three dosing regimens for postoperative analgesia. *Anesthesiology*, **100**(2):395–402.

Porter J M, McCartney C J, Chan V W. (2005). Needle placement and injection posterior to the axillary artery may predict successful infraclavicular brachial plexus block: a report of three cases. *Can J Anaesth*, **52**(1):69–73.

19

Sciatic continuous perineural catheters: proximal and lateral popliteal fossa

Introduction

Use of a continuous perineural catheter is an option for extending anesthesia and analgesia of the lower extremity following sciatic nerve blockade. Patient candidates are often those undergoing painful procedures involving the posterior thigh, leg, foot, and lateral ankle.

Catheter placement may be undertaken wherever the sciatic nerve is approached for blockade prior to separation of the common peroneal and tibial nerves. Ultrasound imaging is a useful tool for identifying the optimal site for catheter placement in addition to providing guidance for catheter insertion and positioning.

Perineural catheter placement is an advanced technique. It is helpful to first gain experience with single-injection sciatic nerve blocking techniques before attempting placement of a continuous catheter with ultrasound.

Ultrasound anatomy review
Distal thigh (lateral popliteal fossa) approach
Orienting structure (distal thigh approach): popliteal artery and biceps femoris muscle (Figures 19.1 and 19.2)

See also Chapter 12: Ultrasound-guided sciatic nerve block: lateral popliteal fossa/distal thigh approach.

Subgluteal approach
Orienting structure (subgluteal approach): the greater trochanter (femur) and fascia (Figure 19.3)

See also Chapter 11: Ultrasound-guided sciatic nerve block: proximal approaches.

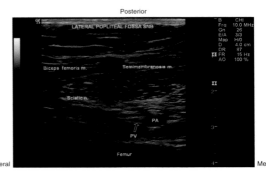

Figure 19.1 Transverse imaging of the sciatic nerve near the popliteal apex. PA = popliteal artery; PV = popliteal vein (partially collapsed).

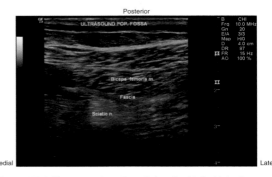

Figure 19.2 Transverse imaging of the distal left thigh above the popliteal space prior to separation of the common peroneal and tibial nerves.

Structures that are required to be identified	Structures that may be seen
Sciatic nerve (tibial nerve/ common peroneal nerve)	Semimembranosis muscle
Popliteal artery	Semitendonosis muscle
Biceps femoris muscle	Popliteal vein
Separation of the sciatic nerve into tibial and common peroneal nerves	Femur
	Fascia

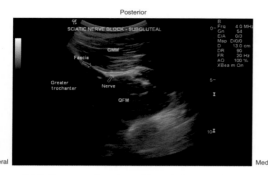

Figure 19.3 Transverse imaging of the sciatic nerve via a subgluteal approach.

Structures that are required to be identified	Structures that may be seen
Greater trochanter of femur	Quadratus femoris muscle
Fascial layer	Ischial tuberosity
Gluteus maximus muscle	

Equipment

- Ultrasound machine
- High-frequency linear array (distal to mid-thigh approach), or low-frequency curved array (proximal thigh approach) ultrasound probe
- Mayo stand or bedside table
- Sterile gown, sterile gloves, hat, and mask
- Sterile skin preparation
- Sterile drape for the procedure site
- Sterile ultrasound controls cover (preferably clear)
- Sterile ultrasound probe sheath with two rubber bands
- Sterile ultrasound gel
- Local anesthetic for skin and subcutaneous infiltration at block needle insertion site
- Blunt-tipped, large-gage, 8-cm Tuohy needle (17-g needle needed to place 19-g catheter; 18-g needle needed to place 20-g catheter)
- Local anesthetic in 10-ml and 20-ml syringes
- Intravascular test dose containing epinephrine
- Sterile, *flexible* catheter with depth markers
- Catheter adapter for syringe/infusion tubing
- Strong skin adhesive (Dermabond® or Histoacryl®) for securing catheter at insertion site
- Less strong adhesive (benzoin or Mastisol®) for securing clear dressing

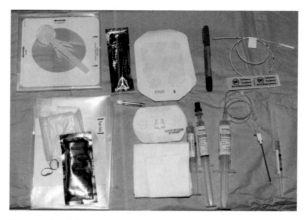

Figure 19.4 Ultrasound-guided perineural cathether kit contents.

- *Transparent* dressing (Tegaderm™ or OpSite™)
- StatLock®
- Illustrated in Figure 19.4

Technique
Technique summary

1. Monitors placed and patient is appropriately positioned and sedated
2. Sterile preparation and drape to procedural site
3. Ultrasound probe and machine are sterilely draped
4. Perform systematic ultrasound scan to find optimal location for catheter insertion
5. Skin wheal is raised
6. Insert Tuohy needle and inject 20 to 30 ml of local anesthetic
7. Disconnect tubing from Tuohy needle
8. Insert catheter through Tuohy needle
9. Remove Tuohy needle while catheter held in place
10. Locate catheter on ultrasound image, then incrementally inject 10 ml of local anesthetic through catheter
11. Pull back on catheter as needed to optimize its position
12. Inject test dose containing epinephrine through catheter
13. Catheter insertion site is sealed with strong skin adhesive
14. Benzoin applied to surrounding skin, catheter is coiled and covered with clear adhesive dressing
15. Catheter hub is secured to the patient with a StatLock® or similar device

171

Patient and equipment preparation

For sciatic catheter placement, patients are placed in the lateral decubitus postion to allow more complete scanning of the sciatic nerve and surrounding structures from distal to proximal positions along the thigh. The ability to scan the length of the sciatic nerve becomes important when determining the optimal site for catheter insertion.

Since continuous catheters require more time to place than single-injection nerve blocks and require the use of larger gauge needles, this procedure may be more uncomfortable and anxiety provoking for the patient. Use of adequate sedation and an assistant, when possible, to monitor the patient and ensure that the patient does not reach into the procedural area and contaminate the field may be beneficial.

Continuous perineural catheters should be placed under strict sterile technique with the physician and his/her assistant wearing a surgical cap, mask, sterile gown, and sterile gloves, as well as sterile covering of the ultrasound transducer and controls. When an assistant is not available, continuous perineural catheters can be placed by an unassisted anesthesiologist (Figure 19.5). The steps taken to prepare the ultrasound machine, probe, and catheter kit by an unassisted anesthesiologist are as follows.

1. Position the patient turned away from the physician and place the ultrasound machine near the head of the patient's bed. Then drape the ultrasound probe over the front of the ultrasound machine, hanging freely (see Figure 15.3).

2. A block table with the sterile equipment for placing a catheter is placed across the patient from the opposite side on which the block will be performed (Figure 19.5).

3. The anesthesiologist should now don the cap, mask, sterile gown, and gloves.

4. Apply a wide sterile preparation to the region of the thigh intended for the procedure, then place a clear, sterile drape over that area (Figure 19.6).

5. Conduction gel is then placed inside the sterile ultrasound probe sheath and the sheath is carefully placed over the hanging probe, then extended over the cord (see Figure 15.4). It is important that the gel is distributed evenly across the tip of the probe to ensure that there are no air bubbles between the probe and the sheath. A rubber band is then placed across the top of the probe to maintain a snug fit. A second rubber band is then applied lower on the probe to ensure that the sheath does not slide while the probe is being handled (see Figure 15.5).

6. With the probe now covered, the ultrasound machine controls are draped with a clear, sterile cover (see Figure 15.6).

7. A small amount of the remaining sterile conduction gel is placed on the patient, so that scanning can now begin.

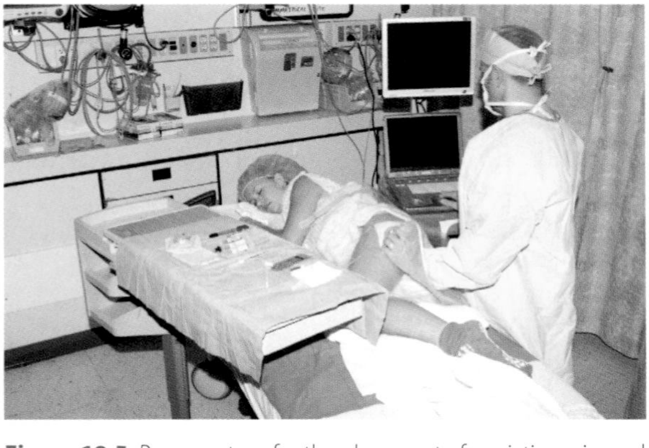

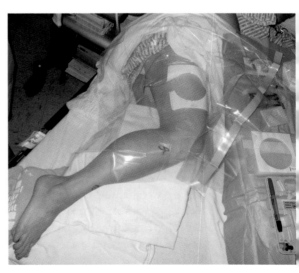

Figure 19.5 Proper set-up for the placement of a sciatic perineural catheter by an unassisted anesthesiologist.

Figure 19.6 Patient draped for the placement of a sciatic perineural catheter.

Scanning
Distal thigh

For procedures of the foot and lateral ankle, a distal approach to the nerve along the thigh near the popliteal apex may be considered.

A high-frequency linear array transducer should be covered as described above for this procedure. Begin the distal scan by placing the transducer transversely along the posterior aspect of the patient's distal thigh near the apex of the popliteal space (Figure 19.7). By convention, the probe should be oriented such that the probe indicator is directed to the patient's right.

Perform a systematic scan of the area, locate orienting structures (e.g., popliteal artery in the apex, biceps femoris muscle), and identify the sciatic nerve (or individual tibial nerve and common peroneal nerve) at this location (Figure 19.8a). Once clearly imaged, follow the nerve or its components proximally along the thigh and note where the common peroneal nerve and tibial nerve converge together.

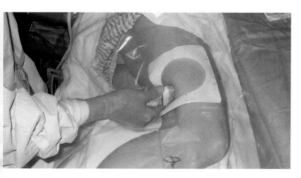

Figure 19.7 Scanning the distal thigh prior to the start of the sciatic nerve catheter procedure.

This location will be most appropriate for distal catheter positioning (Figure 19.8b).

Additional considerations

Distal sciatic nerve catheters may be conveniently placed with the patient kept supine (gapped-supine or leg elevation positioning). A disadvantage of supine positioning for catheter placement, however, is the inability to scan to more proximal points along the thigh (i.e., mid-thigh or higher) should it become necessary for catheter positioning.

In general, consider use of a high-frequency probe for scanning the distal to mid-proximal thigh, and a low-frequency probe for proximal thigh or subgluteal approaches.

Proximal thigh

More proximal positioning (e.g., proximal thigh or subgluteal) of a sciatic nerve catheter may be necessary for procedures involving large (or proximal) portions of the leg or thigh.

For scanning along the upper portion of the thigh, either a low- or high-frequency transducer, prepared with a sterile cover, may be used. As discussed previously, the lower frequency probe should be used if greater tissue penetration is required for imaging.

Begin the proximal scan by orienting the transducer tranversly between the greater trochanter and the ischial tuberosity (Figure 19.9). Perform a systematic scan, moving the probe distally along the thigh while making small probe adjustments (e.g., tilting, rotating, or medial and lateral repositioning) as needed to identify key orienting structures (e.g., greater trochanter, femur, etc.). Once the sciatic nerve is located,

(a)
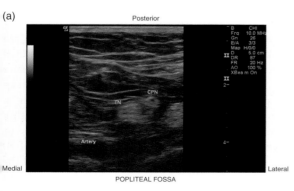

(b)
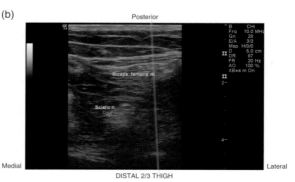

Figures 19.8 (a) and (b) Transverse imaging of the sciatic nerve scanning proximally from the popliteal apex up to the distal thigh to identify the convergence of the common peroneal nerve (CPN) and tibial nerve (TN).

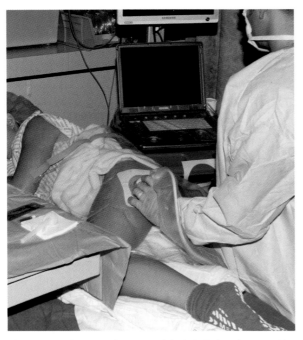

Figure 19.9 Scanning the proximal thigh (subgluteal approach) prior to the start of a sciatic nerve catheter procedure.

follow the nerve to the desired point along the proximal thigh or subgluteal area for catheter insertion (Figure 19.10a, b and c) (See also Chapter 11: Ultrasound-guided sciatic nerve blocks: proximal approaches).

Needle insertion

Having identified the sciatic nerve at an appropriate location for catheter placement, skin infiltration is undertaken on the mid-lateral thigh corresponding to the position of the ultrasound probe. A Tuohy or other blunt-tip needle designed for perineural catheter placement is placed through the skin wheal and advanced in plane with the ultrasound beam.

Recall that along the distal portion of the patient's thigh, the block needle is inserted from a lateral position away from the ultrasound probe being manipulated beneath the patient's leg (as when performing a single-shot lateral popliteal sciatic nerve block with the patient supine; see Chapter 12: Ultrasound-guided sciatic nerve block: lateral popliteal fossa/distal thigh approach) (Figure 19.11). This changes in the middle to proximal portions of the thigh where the needle may be introduced closer to the transducer with the patient in the lateral decubitus position. For the subgluteal approach to the sciatic nerve, the block needle is placed adjacent to the ultrasound probe (Figure 19.12).

As the needle is advanced, look for movement along the corresponding lateral edge of the ultrasound screen. Once under the transducer, and within the course of the ultrasound beam, the needle should appear as a hyperechoic line. Again, do not blindly advance the needle. Advance the tip to a position that ideally pierces the surrounding fascia and is in close proximity to the nerve (Figures 19.13 and 19.14).

Local anesthetic injection and needle repositioning

Prior to catheter placement, local anesthetic is injected around the sciatic nerve through the block needle (Figure 19.15). This bolus injection serves several purposes:

- Injection of local anesthetic and visualization of the anesthetic spread helps to confirm that the tip of the block needle is within the correct fascial plane prior to advancing the catheter through the needle.
- Local anesthetic injection can expand the surrounding tissue and make passage of the catheter easier.
- If the catheter positioning is not optimal, the injection of some local anesthetic prior to catheter placement will give the patient, at the very least, the benefit of a single-injection block.
- Due to the differences in tissue impedance of local anesthetics and the surrounding tissue, a pocket of local anesthetic will make the *visualization* of the perineural catheter easier during positioning.

The needle should be placed in proximity to the nerve to pierce the surrounding fascia, without actually entering the nerve. The nerve itself will appear to be dissected away from the muscle as injection occurs ("hydrodissection") (Figure 19.16). Injections should be performed in 3- to 5-ml increments with small aspirations attempted between injections to ensure the needle tip remains extravascular. The nerve can be approached from above and/or below in order to create a surrounding ring of local anesthetic within which the nerve appears to "float" (i.e., "donut" or "eyeball sign") (Figure 19.17). A bolus volume of 20 to 30 ml is usually sufficient. Following injection, the needle tip is positioned adjacent to the nerve within the fascial pocket of local anesthetic ready for catheter insertion.

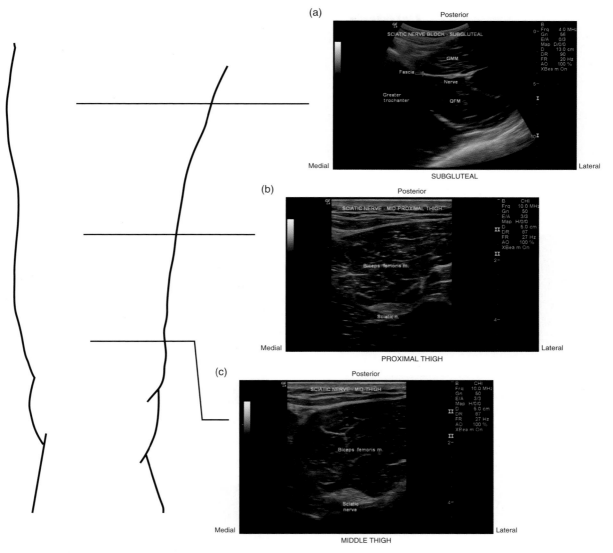

Figures 19.10 (a), (b), and (c) Tranverse images scanning distally along the proximal posterior thigh. GMM = gluteus maximus muscle; QFM = quadratus femoris muscle (Figures b and c imaged with a high-frequency linear array transducer).

Additional considerations

A negative aspiration does not rule out an intravascular injection.

Remain alert to the possibility of intravascular injection if the spread of local anesthetic is not seen, as this may indicate that the local anesthetic is being deposited into a vessel and not perineurally, regardless of a prior negative aspiration.

Whatever total volume of local anesthetic is chosen to be injected, inject all but 10 ml through the needle, saving the last 10 ml to be injected through the catheter itself.

Catheter insertion

Once the fascial plane around the nerve has been expanded with the initial injection of local anesthetic, advance the perineural catheter through the needle into the perineural space created by local anesthetic. Once the catheter is inserted through the Tuohy needle, it will encounter resistance as it exits the tip of the needle. The Tuohy needle must be held in place to facilitate passage of the catheter past its tip. If the needle is not held in place as the catheter is advanced past the tip, pushing the catheter past the

175

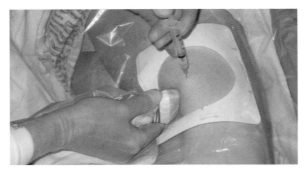

Figure 19.11 Skin and subcutaneous local infiltration at the site of needle insertion (distal thigh/lateral popliteal approach).

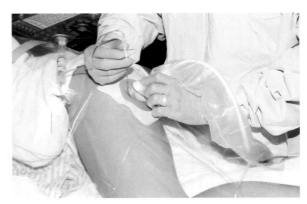

Figure 19.12 Tuohy needle insertion during sciatic catheter placement (subgluteal approach).

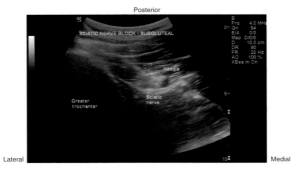

Figure 19.13 Tuohy needle advancement toward the sciatic nerve during sciatic catheter placement (subgluteal approach).

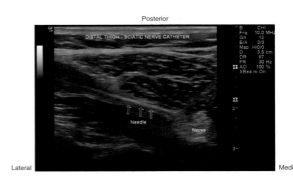

Figure 19.14 Tuohy needle advancement toward the sciatic nerve during sciatic catheter placement (distal thigh/lateral popliteal fossa approach).

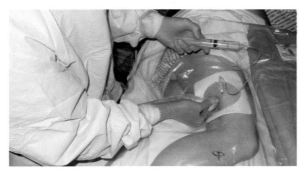

Figure 19.15 Needle insertion prior to local anesthetic injection (distal thigh/lateral popliteal approach).

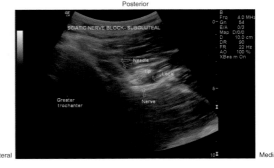

Figure 19.16 Local anesthetic injection around the sciatic nerve prior to sciatic catheter placement (subgluteal approach).

initial resistance at the tip of the needle may cause the needle to move deeper. Too much movement of the needle may cause the catheter to be placed in the wrong position.

The goal for catheter insertion is to insert and advance the catheter under direct ultrasound visualization. Target structures are usually deep enough

that the block needle may be left unsupported while maintaining visualization of the target area with the ultrasound probe (Figures 19.18 and 19.19). To accomplish this, the probe must be properly positioned on the patient as the catheter is advanced

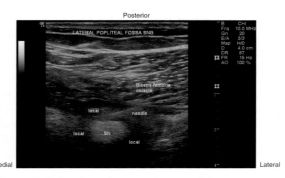

Figure 19.17 Local anesthetic injection around the sciatic nerve prior to sciatic catheter placement (distal thigh/lateral popliteal fossa approach).

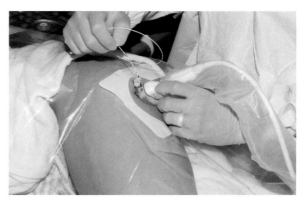

Figure 19.18 Sciatic nerve catheter insertion (subgluteal approach).

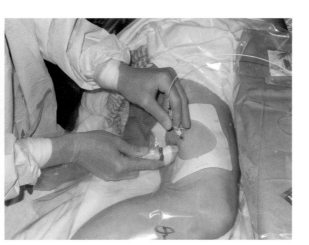

Figure 19.19 Sciatic nerve catheter insertion (distal thigh/lateral popliteal fossa approach.

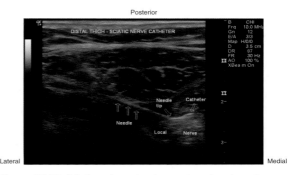

Figure 19.20 Sciatic perineural catheter advancing through a needle under direct ultrasound visualization (distal thigh/lateral popliteal fossa approach).

towards the sciatic nerve. Initially, this may be the most difficult part of placing perineural catheters.

There are two ways to accomplish advancing the catheter under direct visualization by an unassisted anesthesiologist.

1. Once the initial injection of local anesthetic is completed, the ultrasound probe is laid on the sterile drape and the extension tubing is gently disconnected from the Tuohy needle. Next, grasp the Tuohy needle with one hand and advance the catheter just past the tip of the needle with the other hand. As the catheter is advanced, some resistance may be felt as the catheter exits the tip of the needle. Do not advance the catheter if there is too much resistance. If this occurs, rotate the tip of the Tuohy needle or pull the needle back one to two

millimeters and try to advance the catheter again. If these maneuvers fail, gently remove the catheter and inject a few milliliters of local anesthetic through the needle under ultrasound visualization to further expand the tissue, then reinsert the catheter into the needle. Once the catheter has passed the tip of the Tuohy needle, place the probe back on the patient and find the tip of the catheter, which should only be one to two centimeters past the tip of the needle. One may now advance the rest of the catheter through the needle under direct ultrasound visualization (Figure 19.20). With the catheter tip past the tip of the Tuohy needle, the catheter can be advanced without having to hold the needle (Figures 19.18 and 19.19).

2. A more advanced method requires holding the ultrasound probe and Tuohy needle in one hand while advancing the catheter with the other hand. This technique will be most applicable to the

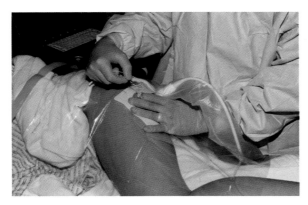

Figure 19.21 Advancement of a perineural catheter through a needle under ultrasound visualization while holding the Tuohy needle.

placement of a sciatic perineural catheter using the *subgluteal* approach. When ready to advance the catheter, hold the ultrasound probe in a manner that will allow one's thumb and first finger to stabilize the ultrasound probe while the Tuohy needle is stabilized between the first and second fingers (Figure 19.21). Another method could be to hold the ultrasound probe in a manner that will allow one's thumb and first finger to grasp the wing of the Tuohy needle while still allowing one to hold the ultrasound probe in the proper position with the remaining fingers. There is now a free hand to remove the extension tubing from the Tuohy needle and advance the catheter through the needle. The Tuohy needle needs to be held firmly between the fingers due to the resistance that is encountered by the catheter as it exits the tip of the needle. This hand positioning may initially feel awkward, especially for practitioners with very small hands. Alternatively, the ultrasound probe can be held with the fingers, but use the thumb or a finger to brace the Tuohy needle by positioning it on the underside of one of the wings of the Tuohy needle, preventing the needle from advancing deeper as the catheter is advanced. Either way, the key point is to stabilize both the ultrasound probe and the needle with one hand. There is now a free hand to remove the extension tubing from the Tuohy needle and advance the catheter through the needle.

It is important to watch the catheter as it is advanced. The optimal distance a catheter is inserted depends on how it behaves during insertion. As the catheter is advanced, it may either travel straight away from the sciatic nerve, without coiling, and poke through the fascial plane containing the local anesthetic from the initial injection or, more likely, begin to coil near the tip of the needle within the space created by the initial local anesthetic bolus. Since the needle tip is near the sciatic nerve, the catheter should coil near the sciatic nerve, within the correct fascial plane. This is the ideal position for the perineural catheter. When the catheter begins to coil, the entire catheter will not be within the ultrasound beam. Therefore, a coiled catheter may only be seen as hyperechoic fragments since only the parts of the coil that cross the ultrasound beam will be visualized. An additional visual confirmation of catheter coiling is movement of tissue within the target fascial plane. Advancing the catheter too far may cause excessive coiling of the catheter, and could potentially lead to knotting of the catheter or entrapment of a nerve. Typically, passing the catheter a distance of 3 to 5 cm past the tip of the needle is sufficient.

Additional considerations

Although coiling of the perineural catheter is ideal, it is not mandatory. Allowing the catheter to coil helps protect against migration away from the target structures.

If the perineural catheter advances straight through the fascial plane without coiling, it may be pulled back, under direct ultrasound visualization, into an acceptable position close to the sciatic nerve after the Tuohy needle has been removed.

Do not pull the catheter back through the needle as this may cause the catheter to shear on the sharp and angled tip of the Tuohy needle. A sheared catheter may break during reinsertion or during removal by the patient.

Confirmation of catheter position

Once the perineural catheter has been placed, hold the catheter in place and slowly back the needle out of the patient over the catheter. When the needle is removed, attach a 10-ml syringe of local anesthetic to the catheter. Next, place the ultrasound probe back on the patient and attempt to visualize the catheter by either tracing the catheter through the soft issue from its insertion site, or by looking for the catheter,

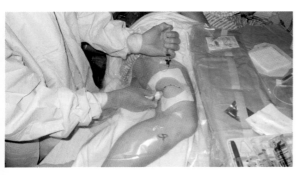

Figure 19.22 Confirming the catheter tip position (distal thigh/lateral popliteal fossa approach).

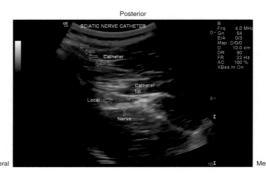

Figure 19.23 Sciatic perineural catheter after positioning (subigluteal approach).

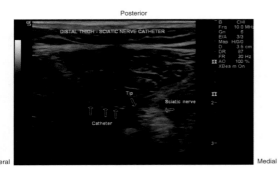

Figure 19.24 Sciatic perineural catheter after positioning (distal thigh approach).

seen as hyperechoic lines, near the sciatic nerve. The 19-gage catheter can be difficult to find after it has been inserted. Although the catheter is larger than the 21-gage needles used for the single-injection technique, it does not always travel in a straight path and therefore only a small portion of it will be within the narrow beam of the ultrasound. It is very difficult to identify the tip of the catheter solely by scanning when the catheter is coiled in the fascial plane. The hydrolocation technique can help identify the catheter tip. To do this, first visualize a portion of the catheter near the sciatic nerve then administer very small, pulsing injections of local anesthetic (or saline) through the catheter (Figure 19.22). There will be an accompanying hypoechoic expansion at the tip of the catheter with every small injection of local anesthetic. If the tip of the catheter has been positioned too far from the sciatic nerve, gently pull back on the catheter, watching it move under direct ultrasound visualization, until the tip is optimally positioned in proximity to the sciatic nerve such that it will continue to provide anesthetic to the target area

as noted by injections through the catheter under ultrasound visualization (Figures 19.23 and 19.24). Here the remainder of the local anesthetic can be injected, and spread of local anesthetic around the sciatic nerve should be observed. At times it may be necessary to remove the catheter completely and restart the procedure if the optimal position is not obtained, or the catheter position fails to be identified.

Just prior to securing the perineural catheter, a test dose containing epinephrine is administered through the catheter to serve as an additional confirmation that the tip of the catheter is not intravascular.

Additional considerations

If the hydrolocation technique is used to find the catheter initially, before a focused scan for the catheter at the sciatic nerve is performed, one may run out of local anesthetic before the tip of the catheter can be identified.

Rhythmic pulsation on the syringe plunger (hydropulsation) attached to the catheter may cause the tip of the catheter to flicker. This may aid in locating the tip of the catheter without using much local anesthetic.

Avoid injecting a large amount of local anesthetic at one time through the catheter without knowing the location of the catheter tip.

A 19-gage catheter, placed through a 17-gage needle, will show injection at the catheter tip much better than a 20-gage catheter.

If difficulty is encountered identifying the location of the catheter tip, a small amount of air (1 or 2 ml) injected through the catheter (while observing the ultrasound screen) may be helpful. The injected air will appear as a hyperechoic artifact originating from the catheter tip.

Securing the catheter at the skin

Once the catheter tip is in the proper location and a negative test dose is confirmed, the catheter may be secured at the skin.

Carefully remove any ultrasound gel from the patient's skin with sterile gauze. A strong skin adhesive or skin glue, such as Dermabond® (Ethicon, Inc., Summerville, NJ, USA) or Histoacryl® (B/BRAUN, Germany; TissueSeal, LLC, Ann Arbor, MI, USA) is applied to the catheter insertion site and allowed to dry. The adhesive should cover an area approximately 1 to 2 cm around the catheter. The purpose of the skin glue is to seal the catheter insertion site, minimizing catheter movement and leakage of local anesthetic during pump infusion, especially when a patient-controlled analgesia (PCA) function is used (Figure 19.25).

A wider area around the catheter insertion site is then painted with a less strong liquid adhesive such as benzoin (Aplicare, Inc., Branford, CT, USA) or Mastisol® (Ferndale Laboratories, Inc., Ferndale, MI, USA) for dressing application. The tail end of the catheter is coiled (to shorten the amount of catheter slack) before placing a transparent adhesive dressing over the entire site. The clear dressing allows the patient to monitor for potential signs of infection (e.g., erythema, drainage, or discharge). After dressing, the catheter is further secured by snapping the injection port into a StatLock® device (C. R. Bard, Inc., Covington, GA, USA), which is placed on the patient adjacent to the catheter site (Figure 19.26).

Additional considerations

Skin glue placed over the catheter insertion site is a key step to prevent leakage of anesthetic and movement of the catheter after it is secured. The less strong adhesives, such as benzoin or Mastisol®, do not form enough of a seal at the catheter insertion site to properly secure or avoid leaking local anesthetic around the catheter.

Authors' clinical practice

- *Infusion regimen:* we use a 0.2% ropivacaine infusion for most of our sciatic perineural catheters, started at 10 ml/hr. A PCA demand option (e.g., 2- to 5-ml bolus every 30 minutes) may be added to the basal infusion.
- Depending on the area to be covered, we usually place sciatic perineural catheters at locations where

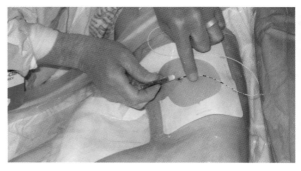

Figure 19.25 Application of a strong skin adhesive to the catheter insertion site. This helps secure the catheter in place and seal the hole made by the large Tuohy needle, preventing leakage of local anesthetic.

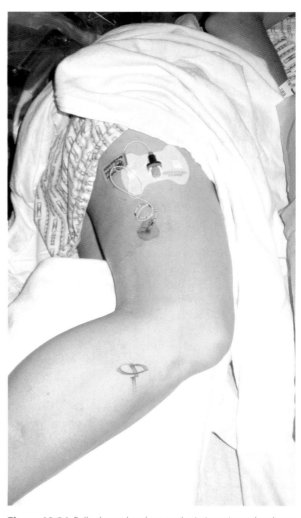

Figure 19.26 Fully dressed and secured sciatic perineural catheter with StatLock®.

the nerve is most easily visualized. Generally, the more proximal the approach, the more challenging it can be to image the nerve, especially in obese patients.

- We generally do not perform anterior sciatic nerve catheters, though this is certainly feasible by the experienced physician.
- We have found that it is not necessary to tunnel the perineural catheter to secure it when the catheter is secured as described above.
- If at any point during the placement of a perineural catheter a vascular puncture occurs we strongly consider placing the catheter at an alternate location or aborting the procedure. Our concerns in this situation include the risk for infection with an indwelling catheter left in a confined space where hematoma formation may occur, and the potential for intravascular leakage of local anesthetic infusing under pressure.
- Catheters are left in place for two to three days depending on the total volume of anesthetic available in the patient's infusion pump. We do not typically leave catheters indwelling beyond three days.
- Patients receiving any sciatic nerve block are at risk for falling following placement of the block. Consideration and discussion should take place with the patient prior to block (and catheter) placement.

Suggested reading

Minville V, Zetlaoui P J, Fessenmeyer C, Benhamou D. (2004). Ultrasound guidance for difficult lateral popliteal catheter insertion in a patient with peripheral vascular disease. *Reg Anesth Pain Med*, **29**(4):368–70.

Sinha A, Chan V W. (2004). Ultrasound imaging for popliteal sciatic nerve block. *Reg Anesth Pain Med*, **29**(2):130–4.

Swenson J D, Bay N, Loose E, *et al.* (2006). Outpatient management of continuous peripheral nerve catheters placed using ultrasound guidance: an experience in 620 patients. *Anesth Analg*, **103**(6):1436–43.

Tsui B C, Finucane B T. (2006). The importance of ultrasound landmarks: a "traceback" approach using the popliteal blood vessels for identification of the sciatic nerve. *Reg Anesth Pain Med*, **31**(5):481–2.

Femoral continuous perineural catheter

Introduction

When the ultrasound single-injection femoral nerve block technique is advanced to a perineural catheter technique, it is able to provide a longer duration of postoperative analgesia for several procedures involving the knee, thigh, and hip. Like the single-injection technique, the placement of a femoral perineural catheter is performed at the inguinal region. Here the perineural catheter can be positioned at the proximal portion of the femoral nerve. Although placement of an ultrasound-guided femoral perineural catheter and an ultrasound-guided single-injection femoral nerve block are similar, advancement to placing a catheter should not occur until proficiency has been achieved with the single-injection technique.

Ultrasound anatomy review

Orienting structure: femoral artery (Figure 20.1)

Equipment

- Ultrasound machine
- High-frequency ultrasound probe
- Mayo stand or bedside table
- Sterile gown, sterile gloves, hat, and mask
- Sterile skin preparation
- Sterile drape for the procedure site
- Sterile ultrasound controls cover (preferably clear)
- Sterile ultrasound probe sheath with two rubber bands
- Sterile ultrasound gel
- Local anesthetic for skin and subcutaneous infiltration at block needle insertion site
- Blunt-tipped, large-gage, 4- to 8-cm, depending on the size of the patient, Tuohy needle (17-gage needle needed to place 19-gage catheter; 18-gage needle needed to place 20-gage catheter)

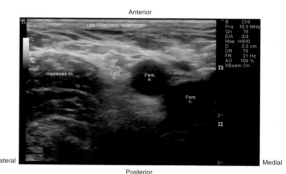

Figure 20.1 Normal femoral ultrasound anatomy near the inguinal crease.

Structures that are required to be identified	Structures that may be seen
Femoral artery	Iliopsoas muscle
Femoral vein	Profunda femoris artery
Femoral nerve	Lateral femoral circumflex artery
	Anomalous vasculature

- Local anesthetic in 10-ml and 20-ml syringes
- Intravascular test dose containing epinephrine
- Sterile, *flexible* catheter with depth markers
- Catheter adapter for syringe/infusion tubing
- Strong skin adhesive, such as Dermabond® (Ethicon, Inc., Summerville, NJ, USA) or Histoacryl® (B/BRAUN, Germany; TissueSeal, LLC, Ann Arbor, MI, USA), for securing catheter at insertion site
- Less strong adhesive, such as benzoin (Aplicare, Inc., Branford, CT, USA) or Mastisol® (Ferndale Laboratories, Inc., Ferndale, MI, USA) for securing clear dressing
- *Clear* Tegaderm™ or OpSite™ dressing

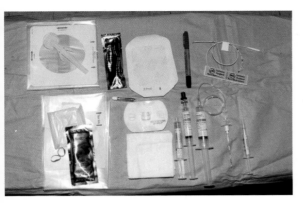

Figure 20.2 Ultrasound-guided perineural catheter kit contents.

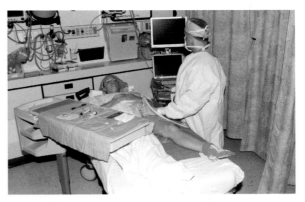

Figure 20.3 Proper set up for the placement of a femoral perineural catheter by an unassisted anesthesiologist.

- StatLock®
- Illustrated in Figure 20.2

Technique
Technique summary

1. Monitors placed and patient is appropriately sedated
2. Sterile preparation and drape to procedural site
3. Ultrasound probe and machine are sterilely draped
4. Perform systematic ultrasound scan to find optimal location for catheter insertion
5. Skin wheal is raised
6. Insert Tuohy needle and inject 20 ml of local anesthetic
7. Disconnect tubing from Tuohy needle
8. Insert catheter through Tuohy needle
9. Remove Tuohy needle while catheter is held in place
10. Locate catheter on ultrasound image, then incrementally inject 10 ml of local anesthetic through catheter
11. Pull back on catheter as needed to optimize its position
12. Inject test dose containing epinephrine through catheter
13. Catheter insertion site is sealed with strong skin adhesive
14. Catheter is coiled and covered with bezoin and a Tegaderm™
15. Catheter hub is secured to the patient with a StatLock® or similar device

Patient and equipment preparation

Since continuous catheters require more time to place than single-injection nerve blocks and require the use of larger gage needles, this procedure may be more uncomfortable and anxiety provoking for the patient. Use of adequate sedation and an assistant, when possible, to monitor the patient and ensure that the patient does not reach into the procedural area and contaminate the field may be beneficial.

Continuous perineural catheters should be placed under strict sterile technique with the physician and his/her assistant, when available, wearing a surgical cap, mask, sterile gown, and sterile gloves, as well as sterile covering of the ultrasound transducer and controls. When an assistant is not available, continuous perineural catheters can be placed by an unassisted anesthesiologist (Figure 20.3). The steps taken to prepare the ultrasound machine, probe, and catheter kit by an unassisted anesthesiologist are as follows.

1. Position the patient and place the ultrasound machine near the head of the patient's bed, as in the single-injection technique, then drape the ultrasound probe over the front of the ultrasound machine, hanging freely (see Figure 15.3).
2. A block table with the equipment for placing a catheter, sterilely laid out on it, is placed across the patient from the opposite side on which the block will be performed (Figure 20.3).
3. The anesthesiologist should now don the cap, mask, sterile gown, and gloves.
4. Apply a wide sterile preparation to the inguinal region, then place a clear, sterile drape over the area.

183

5. Conduction gel is then placed inside the sterile ultrasound probe sheath and the sheath is carefully placed over the hanging probe, then extended over the cord (see Figure 15.4). It is important that the gel is distributed evenly across the tip of the probe to ensure that there are no air bubbles between the probe and the sheath. A rubber band is then placed across the top of the probe to maintain a snug fit. A second rubber band is then applied lower on the probe to ensure that the sheath does not slide while the probe is being handled (see Figure 15.5).

6. With the probe now covered, the ultrasound machine controls are draped with a clear, sterile cover (see Figure 15.6).

7. A small amount of the remaining sterile conduction gel is placed on the patient, so that scanning can now begin.

Scanning

Scanning for perineural catheters is carried out in the same way as for a single-injection femoral nerve block. However, placement of the catheter tip needs to be more precise than that for a single injection. Higher concentrations and larger volumes of local anesthetic used in single-injection blocks can overcome a less precise needle placement. Once the effects of the initial bolus have resolved, the infusion of the local anesthetic from the catheter tip may not reach all the structures affected by the initial bolus of local anesthetic unless positioned optimally. By performing a systematic scan high in the thigh at the inguinal crease, one can identify an ideal position to place the perineural catheter. This should be proximal to the branching of both the profunda femoris and lateral femoral circumflex arteries, and no anomalous vasculature should be in the vicinity of the femoral nerve or in the tissue lateral to the nerve where the large-bore needle needed to place the catheter will pass.

Needle insertion

The needle is inserted and guided *in plane* with the ultrasound beam, just as in a single-injection femoral nerve block. The needle should travel in a lateral to medial direction, posteriorly towards the femoral nerve (Figure 20.4). Make certain to visualize the needle and always be aware of where the needle tip is throughout the procedure. The path of the needle should be aimed just lateral to the femoral nerve, steering the needle around and posterior to the nerve, the same as for a single-injection femoral nerve block.

Needle insertion can also occur away from the lateral edge of the ultrasound probe (Figure 20.5). By doing this, it forces the needle to travel further in the subcutaneous tissue before reaching its target. This will help secure the catheter once the needle has been removed, especially in very skinny patients. Also, inserting the needle away from the edge of the probe forces the use of a shallower needle-insertion angle. Recall that a shallow needle-insertion angle relative to the ultrasound probe will allow for easier visualization of the needle. This will help guide the needle tip to its ideal position.

Insertion of a perineural catheter requires the use of a large-bore needle, relative to the needle used for placement of a single-injection block. Due to their larger diameter, they may present some potential

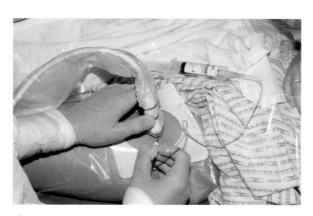

Figure 20.4 Ultrasound and in-plane needle position for the placement of a femoral perineural catheter.

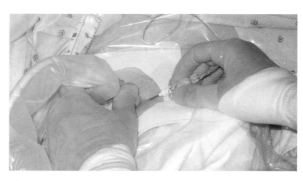

Figure 20.5 Needle insertion lateral from the edge of the ultrasound probe.

problems. First, they often cause more discomfort for the patient, so we recommend not only raising a skin wheal with local anesthetic prior to inserting the large needle, but also infiltrating some of the subcutaneous tissue and iliopsoas muscle with local anesthetic along the potential path of the large needle. Second, the large, blunt-tipped needles used for placement of the catheters can create channels that allow leakage of local anesthetic after the catheter placement. Multiple passes with these large needles will increase the probability of local anesthetic leakage from the targeted area and lead to patient discomfort. If several needle passes are required, do not take the needle out of the skin and create another hole in the skin, but rather redirect the needle in the subcutaneous tissue, deep to the fascia lata, through the same skin hole already created. Multiple holes in the skin can lead to leaking of local anesthetic and wetness under the dressing, which can loosen the dressing and dislodge the catheter. Also, the fascia lata can act as a barrier to keep local anesthetic from leaking into the surrounding subcutaneous tissue, so keeping the needle tip deep to the fascia lata during redirections can minimize the channels for potential leakage of the local anesthetic away from its target structures. Third, large blunt needles can create tears in arteries and veins, which can lead to bleeding and hematomas.

Additional considerations

The most important part of the needle to keep in constant visualization is the needle tip. If the tip is not constantly visualized, one is never certain as to where it is located and what structures it may be penetrating. The only part of the needle that can be visualized is the part that is traveling through the narrow ultrasound beam.

Local anesthetic injection and needle repositioning

Injection through the Tuohy needle prior to placement of the perineural catheter serves several purposes, as follows.

- Injection of local anesthetic and visualization of the spread serves as a confirmation that the location of the needle is within the correct fascial plane, so the catheter should also pass within the correct fascial plane.

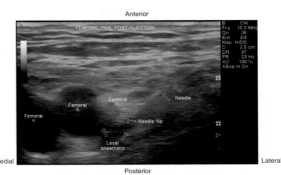

Figure 20.6 Initial injection and spread of local anesthetic through a properly positioned needle prior to femoral perineural catheter placement.

- Local anesthetic injection can expand the surrounding tissue and make passage of the catheter easier.
- If the catheter ends up positioned incorrectly, the injection of some local anesthetic prior to catheter placement will give the patient, at the very least, the benefit of a single-injection block, even if they do not get the benefit of the catheter due to incorrect placement.
- Due to the differences in acoustic impedance of local anesthetics and the surrounding tissue, a pocket of local anesthetic will make the visualization of the needle tip and perineural catheter easier.

Injection of local anesthetic prior to placing a femoral perineural catheter is carried out in the same way as for a single-injection femoral nerve block. With injection of local anesthetic posterior to the femoral nerve, make certain to observe the pattern of local anesthetic spread to confirm positioning of the needle tip within the correct fascial plane. If the needle needs to be redirected to position the tip within the correct fascial plane, or to aid in circumferential spread of the local anesthetic around the femoral nerve, remember to keep the needle tip deep to the fascia lata. After the injection of the full amount of local anesthetic to be deposited through the needle is complete, ensure that the needle tip is positioned just posterior to the femoral nerve (Figure 20.6). This will allow for advancement and coiling of the perineural catheter near the femoral nerve and allow for ideal positioning of the catheter tip.

185

A negative aspiration does not rule out an intravascular injection.

Remain alert to the possibility of intravascular injection if the spread of local anesthetic is not seen, as this may indicate that the local anesthetic is being deposited into a vessel and not perineurally, regardless of a prior negative aspiration.

Whatever total volume of local anesthetic is chosen to be injected, inject all but 10 ml through the needle, saving the last 10 ml to be injected through the catheter itself.

Catheter insertion

Once the catheter is inserted through the Tuohy needle, it will encounter resistance as it exits the tip of the needle. The Tuohy needle must be held in place to facilitate passage of the catheter past its tip. If the needle is not held in place as the catheter is advanced past the tip, pushing the catheter past the initial resistance at the tip of the needle may cause the needle to move deeper. Too much movement of the needle may cause the catheter to be placed in the wrong position.

The goal for catheter insertion is to insert and advance the catheter under direct ultrasound visualization (Figure 20.7). To accomplish this, the probe must be properly positioned on the patient as the catheter is advanced towards the femoral nerve. Initially, this may be the most difficult part of placing perineural catheters.

There are two ways to accomplish advancing the catheter under direct visualization by an unassisted anesthesiologist.

1. Once the initial injection of local anesthetic is completed, the ultrasound probe is laid on the sterile drape and the extension tubing is gently disconnected from the Tuohy needle. Next, grasp the Tuohy needle with one hand and advance the catheter just past the tip of the needle with the other hand (Figure 20.8). As the catheter is advanced, some resistance may be felt as the catheter exits the tip of the needle. Do not advance the catheter if there is too much resistance. If this occurs, rotate the tip of the Tuohy needle or pull the needle back one to two millimeters and try to advance the catheter again. If these maneuvers fail, gently remove the catheter and inject a few milliliters of local anesthetic through the needle under ultrasound visualization to further expand the tissue, then reinsert the catheter into the needle. Once the catheter has passed the tip of the Tuohy needle, place the probe back on the patient and find the tip of the catheter, which should only be one to two centimeters past the tip of the needle. One may now advance the rest of the catheter through the needle under direct ultrasound visualization (Figure 20.7). With the catheter tip past the tip of the Tuohy needle, the catheter can be advanced without having to hold the needle.

2. A more advanced method requires holding the ultrasound probe and Tuohy needle in one hand while advancing the catheter with the other hand. When ready to advance the catheter, hold the ultrasound probe in a manner that will allow one's thumb and first finger to grasp the wing of the Tuohy needle while still allowing one to hold the ultrasound probe in the proper position with the

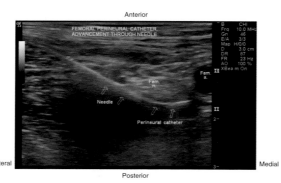

Figure 20.7 Femoral perineural catheter advancing through a needle under direct ultrasound visualization.

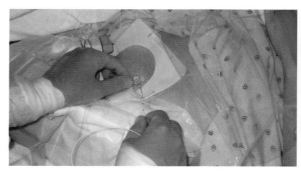

Figure 20.8 The Tuohy needle is grasped in one hand while the other advances the catheter.

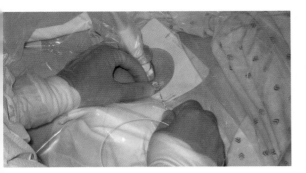

Figure 20.9 Advancement of a perineural catheter through a needle under ultrasound visualization while holding the Tuohy needle.

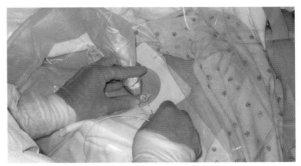

Figure 20.10 Advancement of a perineural catheter through a needle under ultrasound visualization while bracing the Tuohy needle.

remaining fingers. There is now a free hand to remove the extension tubing from the Tuohy needle and advance the catheter through the needle (Figure 20.9). The Tuohy needle needs to be held firmly between the finger tips due to the resistance that is encountered by the catheter as it exits the tip of the needle. This hand positioning may initially feel awkward, especially for practitioners with very small hands. Alternatively, the ultrasound probe can be held with the fingers, but use the thumb to brace the Tuohy needle by positioning it on the underside of one of the wings of the Tuohy needle, preventing the needle from advancing deeper as the catheter is advanced (Figure 20.10). Either way, the key point is to stabilize both the ultrasound probe and the needle with one hand. There is now a free hand to remove the extension tubing from the Tuohy needle and advance the catheter through the needle.

It is important to watch the catheter as it is advanced. The optimal distance a catheter is inserted depends on how it behaves during insertion. As the catheter is advanced, it may either travel straight away from the femoral nerve, without coiling, and poke through the fascial plane containing the local anesthetic from the initial injection or, more likely, begin to coil near the tip of the needle within the space created by the initial local anesthetic bolus. Since the needle tip is near the femoral nerve, the catheter should coil near the femoral nerve, within the correct fascial plane. This is the ideal position for the perineural catheter. When the catheter begins to coil, the entire catheter will not be within the ultrasound beam. Therefore, a coiled catheter may only be seen as

hyperechoic fragments since only the parts of the coil that cross the ultrasound beam will be visualized. An additional visual confirmation of catheter coiling is movement of tissue within the target fascial plane. Advancing the catheter too far may cause excessive coiling of the catheter, and could potentially lead to knotting of the catheter or entrapment of a nerve. Typically, passing the catheter a distance of 3 to 5 cm past the tip of the needle is sufficient.

Additional considerations
Although coiling of the perineural catheter is ideal, it is not mandatory. Allowing the catheter to coil helps protect against migration away from the target structures.
If the perineural catheter advances straight through the fascial plane without coiling, it may be pulled back, under direct ultrasound visualization, into an acceptable position close to the femoral nerve after the Tuohy needle has been removed.
Do not pull the catheter back through the needle as this may cause the catheter to shear on the sharp and angled tip of the Tuohy needle. A sheared catheter may break during reinsertion or during removal by the patient.

Confirmation of catheter position

Once the perineural catheter has been placed, hold the catheter in place and slowly back the needle out of the patient over the catheter (Figure 20.11). When the needle is removed, attach a 10-ml syringe of local anesthetic to the catheter. Next, place the ultrasound probe back on the patient and attempt to visualize the catheter by either tracing the catheter through the soft

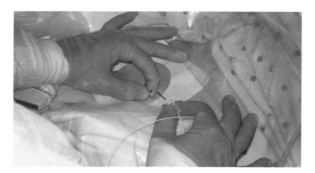

Figure 20.11 Removing the needle from a patient while the catheter remains in place.

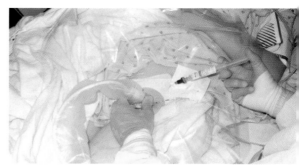

Figure 20.12 Injection through a catheter to locate the tip.

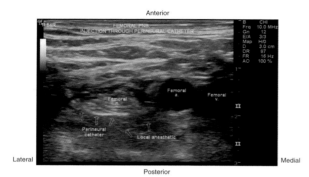

Figure 20.13 Ideal position of a femoral perineural catheter tip posterior to the femoral nerve.

issue from its insertion site, or by looking for the catheter, seen as hyperechoic lines, near the femoral nerve. The 19-gage catheter can be difficult to find after it has been inserted. Although the catheter is larger than the 22-gage needle used for the single-injection technique, it does not always travel in a straight path and therefore only a small portion of it will be within the narrow beam of the ultrasound. It is very difficult to identify the tip of the catheter solely by scanning when the catheter is coiled in the fascial plane. The hydrolocation technique can help identify the catheter tip. To do this, first visualize a portion of the catheter near the femoral nerve then administer very small, pulsing injections of local anesthetic (or saline) through the catheter (Figure 20.12). There will be an accompanying hypoechoic expansion at the tip of the catheter with every small injection of local anesthetic. If the tip of the catheter has been positioned too far from the posterior side of the femoral nerve, gently pull back on the catheter, watching it move under direct ultrasound visualization, until the

tip is optimally positioned posterior to the femoral nerve (Figure 20.13). Here the remainder of the local anesthetic can be injected, and spread of local anesthetic around the femoral nerve should be observed. At times it may be necessary to remove the catheter completely and restart the procedure if the optimal position is not obtained, or the catheter position fails to be identified.

Just prior to securing the perineural catheter, a test dose containing epinephrine is administered through the catheter to serve as an additional confirmation that the tip of the catheter is not intravascular.

Additional considerations

If the hydrolocation technique is used to find the catheter initially, before a focused scan for the catheter at the femoral nerve is performed, one may run out of local anesthetic before the tip of the catheter can be identified.

Rhythmic pulsation on the syringe plunger (hydropulsation) attached to the catheter may cause the tip of the catheter to flicker. This may aid in locating the tip of the catheter without using much local anesthetic.

Avoid injecting a large amount of local anesthetic at one time through the catheter without knowing the location of the catheter tip.

A 19-gage catheter, placed through a 17-gage needle, will show injection at the catheter tip much better than a 20-gage catheter.

If one is having significant difficulty identifying the location of the catheter and/or its tip, one can inject a small amount of air through the catheter while watching the ultrasound screen. The air should show up as a hyperechoic artifact that originates from the catheter tip.

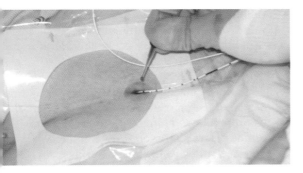

Figure 20.14 Application of a strong skin adhesive to the catheter insertion site. This helps secure the catheter in place and seal the hole made by the large Tuohy needle, preventing leakage of local anesthetic.

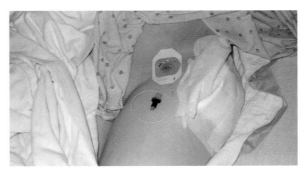

Figure 20.15 Catheter site is dressed with a less strong skin adhesive and a small, clear adhesive dressing.

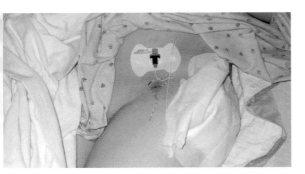

Figure 20.16 Fully dressed and secured femoral perineural catheter with StatLock®.

Securing and dressing the catheter at the skin

Once the catheter tip is in the proper location and a negative test dose is confirmed, the catheter may be secured at the skin.

Carefully remove any ultrasound gel from the patient's skin with sterile gauze. Strong skin adhesive or skin glue, such as Dermabond® (Ethicon, Inc., Summerville, NJ, USA) or Histoacryl® (B/BRAUN, Germany; TissueSeal, LLC, Ann Arbor, MI, USA) is applied to the catheter insertion site and allowed to dry (Figure 20.14). The adhesive should cover an area approximately 1 to 2 cm around the catheter. The purpose of the skin glue is to seal the catheter insertion site, minimizing catheter movement and leakage of local anesthetic during pump infusion, especially when a patient-controlled analgesia (PCA) function is used.

A wider area around the catheter insertion site is then painted with a less strong liquid adhesive, such as benzoin (Aplicare, Inc., Branford, CT, USA) or Mastisol® (Ferndale Laboratories, Inc., Ferndale, MI, USA) for dressing application. The tail end of the catheter is coiled (to shorten the amount of catheter slack) before placing a transparent adhesive dressing over the entire site (Figure 20.15). The clear dressing allows the patient to monitor for potential signs of infection (e.g., erythema, drainage, or discharge). After dressing, the catheter is further secured by snapping the injection port into a StatLock® (C. R. Bard, Inc., Covington, GA, USA), which is placed on the patient adjacent to the catheter site (Figure 20.16).

Additional considerations

Skin glue placed over the catheter insertion site is a key step to prevent leakage of anesthetic and movement of the catheter after it is secured. The less strong adhesives, such as benzoin or Mastisol®, do not form enough of a seal at the catheter insertion site to properly secure or avoid leaking local anesthetic around the catheter.

Authors' clinical practice

- *Infusion regimen for knee procedures:* we have found the most success using 0.1% to 0.2% ropivacaine at a higher basal infusion rate of 10 ml/hr plus a PCA of 2 to 5 ml every 30 to 60 minutes. With our current pump volumes of 550 ml, this typically allows the patient to have good analgesia from the perineural catheter for approximately 2 to 2½ days after discharge from the PACU.

- We typically use 0.1% ropivacaine for surgical procedures in which there is early, aggressive physical therapy and/or ambulation when the knee is not reinforced to prevent buckling. An example of a common surgical procedure for this is an anterior cruciate ligament (ACL) repair.

- We typically use 0.2% ropivacaine for all other surgical procedures of the knee where either the patient will be non-ambulatory or non-weight bearing during the time period when the catheter will infuse (e.g., knee multi-ligament repair or microfracture repair) or the patient will be wearing some type of knee immobilization device immediately after surgery, preventing the leg from buckling during physical therapy (e.g., total knee arthroplasty).

- We have found the difference in analgesia between 0.1% and 0.2% ropivacaine as an infusate to be minimal except for more involved procedures such as total knee arthroplasties, which tend to be very painful, and the patient's pain is much better controlled with 0.2% ropivacaine.

- In most cases, we have seen a significant difference in preservation of motor function when 0.1% ropivacaine is used as the infusate instead of 0.2%.

- *Infusion regimen for hip procedures:* We have found the most success using 0.1% ropivacaine at a higher basal infusion rate of 10 ml/hr plus a PCA of 2 to 5 ml every 30 to 60 minutes. With our current pump volumes of 550 ml, this typically allows the patient to have good analgesia from the perineural catheter for approximately 2 to 2½ days after discharge from the PACU.

  - We use 0.1% ropivacaine because the patients that undergo hip surgeries do not typically wear a knee support on the operative side to prevent the leg from buckling during physical therapy or ambulation, so preservation of motor function is important.

  - In general, procedures of the hip tend to be less painful than procedures of the knee. We have found the difference in analgesia between 0.1% and 0.2% ropivacaine as an infusate after hip procedures (e.g., total hip arthroplasties or hip arthroscopies) to be minimal.

- The total dose of our initial injection for placement of the perineural catheters is the same as when a single-injection nerve block is performed, except that the last 10 ml are injected through the catheter after it has been positioned.

- Although sepsis or untreated bacteremia is considered a relative contraindication to placing a single-injection nerve block, we consider it to be an absolute contraindication to placing a perineural catheter.

- If a vascular puncture occurs at any point during the placement of a perineural catheter we abort the procedure. Our concerns in this situation include risk for infection with an indwelling catheter left in a confined space with a surrounding hematoma, and potential for intravascular leakage of local anesthetic being continuously infused under pressure.

- For our total knee and hip arthroplasty patients, as well as hip arthroscopy patients, we typically place the femoral perineural catheter postoperatively, immediately after the patient arrives at the PACU. This avoids the catheter from potentially being located in the sterile preparation or fluoroscopy field, or having the catheter dislodged intraoperatively.

- In order to have the highest success with postoperative pain relief for patients undergoing hip procedures, it is critical that the perineural catheter be placed as proximal in the thigh as possible, usually in the region between the inguinal crease and the inguinal ligament.

- We have found that it is not necessary to tunnel the perineural catheter to secure it, as long as the steps described in this chapter are performed.

- Patients receiving a femoral continuous peripheral nerve block are at risk for falling throughout the duration of their catheter infusion. Consideration and discussion of this fall risk should take place with the patient prior to sedation and placement of the catheter.

Suggested reading

De Ruyter M L, Brueilly K E, Harrison B A, *et al.* (2006). A pilot study on continuous femoral perineural catheter for analgesia after total knee arthroplasty: the effect on physical rehabilitation and outcomes. *J Arthroplasty*, 21(8):1111–17.

Ilfeld B M, Le L T, Meyer R S, *et al.* (2008). Ambulatory continuous femoral nerve blocks decrease time to discharge readiness after tricompartmental total knee arthroplasty: a randomized, triple-masked, placebo-controlled study. *Anesthesiology*, 108(4):703–13.

Shum C F, Lo N N, Yeo S J, *et al.* (2009). Continuous femoral nerve block in total knee arthroplasty: immediate and two-year outcomes. *J Arthroplasty*, 24(2):204–9.

Index

191

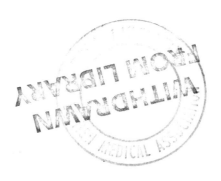